SUPER SOY
THE MIRACLE BEAN

Also by the Author

A Consumer's Guide to Medicines in Food

A Consumer's Dictionary of Medicines

A Consumer's Dictionary of Cosmetics Ingredients

A Consumer's Dictionary of Food Additives

A Consumer's Dictionary of Household, Yard,
and Office Chemicals

Poisons in Your Food

Ageless Aging

Cancer-Causing Agents

How to Reduce Your Medical Bills

SUPER SOY

THE
MIRACLE BEAN

Includes a Cookbook of 50 Soy Recipes

Ruth Winter, M.S.

CROWN TRADE PAPERBACKS   NEW YORK

Copyright © 1996 by Ruth Winter

Published by Crown Trade Paperbacks, 201 East 50th Street, New York, New York 10022. Member of the Crown Publishing Group.

Random House, Inc. New York, Toronto, London, Sydney, Auckland

CROWN TRADE PAPERBACKS and colophon are trademarks of Crown Publishers, Inc.

Printed in the United States of America

Soybean drawing by Jennifer Harper

Design by June Bennett-Tantillo

Library of Congress Cataloging-in-Publication Data is available upon request

ISBN 0-517-88734-7

10   9   8   7   6   5   4   3   2   1

First Edition

Contents

Introduction

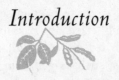

The Cinderella Bean

Within the tiny soybean—about a quarter inch in size—lie many extremely powerful substances that recent scientific studies have found may:

- Lower cholesterol
- Fight cancer
- Reduce blood pressure
- Protect the heart
- Regulate blood sugar
- Ease menstrual and menopausal symptoms
- Promote healthy bowel function
- Nourish babies and adults suffering from allergies
- Strengthen bones

A report in the prestigious *New England Journal of Medicine* on August 3, 1995, created quite a stir among professionals and consumers. Dr. James Anderson and his colleagues at the University of Kentucky and the Veterans Affairs Medical Center in Kentucky analyzed thirty-eight carefully performed studies of the effect of soy protein on blood cholesterol in patients. The Kentuckians concluded that as little as twenty-five to forty-seven grams (about ⅛ to

¼ cup) each day of soybean protein significantly lowered cholesterol. Less publicized but equally as exciting to researchers have been recent reports that nonnutritive substances in soybeans, such as genistein and daizein, show activity against breast, prostate, leukemia, and melanoma (deadly skin) cancers.

The health benefits of the soybean (*Glycine max*) is not news to the Chinese. They call the soybean *ta-tou*—which means "greater bean"—and have been using it for thousands of years as a medicine as well as food. The soybean has been so essential to Chinese civilization in fact that it is considered one of the five sacred grains (the others being rice, barley, wheat, and millet). Legend has it that around 1500 B.C., Yu Xi-ong and Gong Gang-shi—who were either bandits or warlords—became lost in a desert in northern China. They survived on the "peas" of a hitherto unknown plant, believed to be the soybean's wild ancestor, a rambling vine (*Glycine ussuriensis*). Some centuries after Yu Xi-ong and Gong Gang-shi were long gone, the soybean became a *cultigen,* a species created by cultivation.

Miso, fermented soybean paste, appeared in Japan in the 600s as a treat for the shogun and his imperial household. The first mention of soybeans in Japanese literature occurred in 712 A.D. in a book of mythology, *Kojiki.*

The introduction of soybeans into the United States in 1804 was also quite a tale. Clipper ships from China used soybeans as inexpensive ballast. Upon arrival, the beans were tossed overboard. Entrepreneurial—or very hungry—American farmers took the discarded beans and planted them in tillable soil. By the turn of the century, hundreds of farmers in the United States were utilizing the almost effortlessly grown and easily harvested soybeans as a feed crop for cattle.

During the chaos of the Civil War, soybeans found a new niche. They were roasted and used in place of scarce coffee beans. Nearly forty years later, the son of a slave, George Washington Carver, who was born during the Civil War, laid the foundation for today's soybean bonanza. A chemist who did so much for peanut production, Carver discovered that soybeans were also a valuable source of protein and oil. The vegetable oil industry became interested in the soybean's potential. The soybean-processing facilities really began to blossom in the early 1920s and gave cultivation of the Cinderella bean a great impetus.

In 1929, soybean pioneer William J. Morse trekked across China and gathered more than 10,000 varieties of the plant for American researchers to study. A large cooperative program involving both U.S. and Canadian researchers then began to develop improved soybean varieties that produced higher yields of oil.

In the 1940s, soybean farming in North America really burgeoned because the soybean fields in China, a major supplier of soybeans to the world at that time, were devastated by World War II and by China's own civil war. With the new varieties of soybeans developed by American researchers and the greatly expanded sales opportunities, the United States became the world's leading producer and now holds 60 percent of the market. The soybean is also a top crop in the United States itself, ranking only behind corn and wheat. The rapid increase in production in such a relatively short period of time is one of the most striking developments in U.S. agricultural history.

The two basic products of the soybean today are oil and protein meal. In the United States, more than 90 percent of the oil is consumed as margarine, shortening, mayonnaise, and salad oils. It is an ingredient in bakery products, frozen desserts, infant formula, baby food, meat extenders, and coffee creamers. Soy is often the "vegetable" in vegetable oils. Soy shows up in pancake mix, barbecue sauce, bouillon, croutons, and syrup for sundaes.

Ten percent of the oil is used in industrial products such as paint, varnish, linoleum, and rubber fabrics. Soybean meal is the major source of the protein supplement used in livestock feeds, which utilizes 98 percent of the total meal produced.

So it is easy to understand that soybeans are a valuable crop, but what about their food and health values for us?

We could not survive on soybeans alone, but if we are ever lost on a desert island, we should be sure to have some with us. Soybeans contain all three of the macronutrients we need for good nutrition—protein, carbohydrate, and fat—as well as dietary fiber, vitamins, and minerals, including calcium, folic acid, and iron. They also contain a number of nonnutrients that, as you will read in this book, are useful in preventing and perhaps treating a number of major human ills.

The constant construction and destruction of proteins in the body means that a continual supply of amino acids, the building blocks of protein, must be made available in the diet. *Soybeans are the only vegetable food that contain complete protein.* The amino acid pattern of soy protein is essentially equivalent in quality to that of meat, milk, and eggs. In fact, soybeans contain:

- 1½ times as much protein as cheese
- Twice as much as meat or fish
- Three times as much as eggs
- Eleven times as much as milk

The soybean is also a much less expensive source of high-quality protein. Soy protein is very efficiently produced and is more than twenty-five times as efficient per acre of land compared with beef and five times more efficient than wheat.

The once cast-off bean will soon become of even greater value. As more and more healthful substances are isolated from it, soybean *nutraceuticals* will be created. A *nutraceutical* is any substance that may be considered a food or part of a food and provides medical or health benefits, including the prevention and treatment of disease. Such products may range from isolated nutrients, dietary supplements, and diets to genetically engineered "designer" foods, herbal products, and processed foods such as cereals, soups, and beverages.

The term was coined by Stephen L. DeFelice, M.D., chairman of The Foundation for Innovation in Medicine, to give the wide-ranging field an identity because it extends from observing what chimpanzees eat when they don't feel well to creating superfoods through biotechnology. At present, there is no legal term or definition in the United States for products emanating from this field of research.

As you will read in this book, however, there is no doubt that nutraceuticals are being found in the easily grown and harvested abundant soybean. Soy products that are substitutes for meat and fatty foods are already contributing to more healthy diets. Genetic engineers are experimenting with a "gene gun" to shoot foreign genes into a soybean to make it into an edible vaccine. The use of soy and its derivatives as medications has opened up a whole new horizon for this tiny Cinderella bean.

Chapter 1

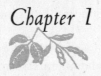

How Soy Protects the Heart and Blood Vessels

The recognition that soybeans could significantly combat artery-clogging cholesterol is really not new. As long ago as 1909, Russian scientists postulated that vegetable proteins could reduce coronary artery disease and in 1967, Robert E. Hodges, M.D., then of the University of Iowa Medical School, carried out a soybean-cholesterol study in a maximum security prison ward. Dr. Hodges reported in the *American Journal of Clinical Nutrition* that there was a significant drop in blood cholesterol in six prisoners with high cholesterol after a four-week, Asian-type soybean-laced diet. And since 1971, Italian scientist Cesare R. Sirtori, M.D. and his colleagues at the Institute of Pharmacological Science and the University of Milan have been reporting success in lowering cholesterol and blood fats in both children and adults with soy protein.

Cholesterol is a fatlike, waxy substance found in animal tissue. It is present in foods from animal sources such as whole milk dairy products, meat, fish, poultry, and egg yolks. An estimated 400 to 500 milligrams or more of cholesterol is ingested each day in the average American diet. Cholesterol is also produced in the body—primarily by the

liver—in varying amounts but usually about 1000 milligrams a day.

Cholesterol isn't all bad. In fact, it is essential for
producing new cells and manufacturing certain hormones.
It is delivered throughout our bodies by tiny packages
made of fat and protein called lipoproteins. Lipoproteins
are flat, disclike particles produced in the liver and intestines and released into the bloodstream. There are basically two major types, *high-density lipoproteins* (HDL)
and low-density lipoproteins (LDL). It is believed that
HDL picks up cholesterol and brings it back to our livers
for reprocessing. Some researchers believe that HDL may
also remove excess cholesterol from fat-gorged cells, possibly even those in artery walls. Because HDL clears cholesterol out of the system and high levels of it are associated
with decreased risk of heart disease, HDL is often called
"good cholesterol." LDL, on the other hand, is considered
"bad" because it deposits fatty junk along artery walls as it
travels from the liver to the cells of the body.

The National Institutes of Health's National Cholesterol Education Program Guidelines say:

- Total cholesterol should be below 200 milligrams
  per deciliter of blood (mg/dl).
- LDL should be below 100 mg/dl of blood if we
  have heart disease or two or more risk factors
  (such as smoking and obesity). It can be 130 if we
  have no coronary artery disease or risk factors.
- HDL cholesterol should be 45 mg/dl or higher for
  men and 55 mg/dl or higher for women.

It is not only the total amount of cholesterol in our
blood that is important but how much of each type of
lipoprotein package we have carting our cholesterol
around.

University of Milan's Dr. Sirtori and his colleagues fed a diet based on vegetable protein—in most cases, textured vegetable protein (TVP) made from soy—to 1000 patients and found an 8 to 25 percent reduction in total blood cholesterol and 15 to 20 percent in LDL cholesterol. Dr. Sirtori contends the soybean diet after a while raised the good HDL cholesterol and not only halted the progression of arterial heart disease but reversed it to an extent.

The soybean diet even counteracted the effects of a high-fat diet. When Dr. Sirtori's group added 500 milligrams of cholesterol—the amount in a couple of eggs—to patients' diets, the soybeans apparently overcame the egg's cholesterol-raising potential and still kept blood cholesterol down. Once the blood cholesterol was lowered, the patients went back to their regular diets but ate at least six meals in a week using textured soybean protein; their cholesterol levels still remained low during the two years they were followed.

At the First International Symposium on the Role of Soy in Preventing and Treating Chronic Disease held in Mesa, Arizona, February 20–23, 1994, Dr. Sirtori pointed out that problems occurred in the soy-cholesterol studies in the past because of poor compliance but now with new, more palatable products such as soy cheeses and yogurts, following a soy-laced diet will be easier for Westerners.

A year and a half after that first symposium was held, public interest was highly aroused by a study published in the August 3, 1995, issue of the *New England Journal of Medicine* by University of Kentucky researchers.

Protein Technologies International, which markets soy protein, the United Soybean Board, and the American Soybean Association had given $5000 in 1993 to a team headed by James W. Anderson, M.D., professor of medicine and nutrition at the University of Kentucky. Dr. Anderson, a member of the Protein Technologies advisory group, and his colleagues did not treat patients directly, but instead analyzed the results of thirty-eight well-controlled clinical studies done over the past seventeen years involving 730 volunteers. The Kentuckians used a computer to, in effect, standardize the thirty-eight studies. The result of that meta-analysis was a conclusion that people who added soy protein to their diet lowered the level of the "bad" LDL cholesterol by about 13 percent but didn't show a drop in "good" HDL cholesterol. Those who ingested forty-seven grams of soy protein a day had cholesterol levels drop 9.3 percent a month. However, the effects were significant only for those who already had at least moderately elevated cholesterol just as Iowa's Dr. Hodges and Italy's Dr. Sirtori had reported earlier.

One of the studies evaluated in the Kentuckians' meta-analysis was done at the University of Illinois College of Medicine at Urbana-Champaign and the Veterans Affairs Medical Center, Danville, Illinois. Dr. John Erdman, Jr., who was a researcher in the investigation, studied the effects of soy protein consumption with and without fiber on the blood fats of twenty-six men with mildly elevated cholesterol. Four different dietary treatments were conducted:

- A diet including fifty grams of protein and twenty grams of dietary fiber from soy flour
- A diet including isolated soy protein and soy fiber
- A diet including isolated soy protein and cellulose
- A diet including nonfat dry milk

All the subjects were also on the American Heart Association's prescribed low-cholesterol, low-fat diet. The results were reported in the *American Journal of Clinical Nutrition* in 1993 by Dr. Susan Potter, Dr. Erdman, and their colleagues at the University of Illinois.

In an interview with the author, Dr. Erdman said that the University of Illinois data indicates that people with elevated blood cholesterol can benefit by incorporating small amounts of soybean protein into their diets. The soybean products used in their study were incorporated into conventional bakery products (see pages 106–107), were well accepted by the subjects, and could be added to a typical American diet.

"You don't have to give up meat and dairy products altogether," he said, "but substitute soy protein for twenty-five grams or more of animal protein."

He said the men in the study ate all meals at the Veterans Hospital. They ate a variety of baked goods containing soy. They also ate some meat and dairy, but all followed the American Heart Association's recommended dietary regimen except that 50 percent of their protein intake was soy protein.

The result was that the men who consumed the soy protein and fiber—at twenty to twenty-five grams per day—had a reduction of total cholesterol by 12 percent and LDL (the "bad" cholesterol) by 11.5 percent compared to the controls who did not partake of the soy protein.

This indicates that it was not just the replacement of protein from meat and dairy products that lowered the cholesterol but the addition of the soy, Dr. Erdman said.

A similar study conducted in 1995 in the same manner with postmenopausal women by University of Illinois researchers also showed similar results. The women's cholesterol was lowered by soy protein.

What is it in the soybean that lowers cholesterol and may have other beneficial effects on our hearts and arteries? No one is quite sure, but there are a number of substances in the bean that researchers feel may be responsible.

FULL OF FIBER

It has been shown in other research that certain forms of fiber such as that found in soybeans play a part in lowering cholesterol. Although not fully understood, these soluble fibers move through the small intestine and interfere either with the absorption or the metabolism of cholesterol. Not all fiber is alike. Insoluble dietary fiber is thought to be mainly a bulking agent, increasing stool weight and decreasing transit time. Soybeans contains some of these such as cellulose and lignin. They also contain soluble fibers (about 30 percent) such as gums and pectins that have been shown to decrease serum cholesterol in laboratory studies.

THE ESKIMO SECRET—OMEGA-3 FATTY ACIDS

Fatty acids are the basic chemical units of fat. They can be *saturated, monounsaturated,* or *polyunsaturated,* depending on how many hydrogen atoms they hold. All dietary fats are mixtures of these three types of fatty acids, but they vary in the amount of each they contain. *Polyunsaturated fatty acids,* found mainly in fat from plants, tend to lower blood cholesterol levels while *saturated fatty acids,* found mostly in meat and dairy products but also in some vegetable oils, tend to raise it. Soybeans are high in *polyunsaturated fatty acids* and are a particularly good source of omega-3 fatty acids. Omega-3 is the substance also found in fish that has been credited with keeping Eskimos heart-healthy despite their high-fat diet, according to studies by Danish and University of Chicago researchers. About 62 percent of the oil in soybeans is unsaturated fatty acids and 23 percent monounsaturated, which also does not raise cholesterol, according to the latest research.

LECITHIN AND VITAMIN E

Soybeans are also a good source of lecithin (from the Greek, meaning "egg yolk"). They also have very small amounts of vitamin E. In fact, vitamin E was first identified in soy, according to Dr. James Clark of the Henkel Corporation in LaGrant, Illinois. Henkel is the world's largest manufacturer of natural source vitamin E. Both lecithin and vitamin E are natural antioxidants, and folk medicine practitioners have long used them to lower cholesterol.

Researchers now believe that oxidation of LDL cholesterol is the main culprit in the progressive hardening and blocking of the arteries known as atherosclerosis. Soy milk (see page 89) was shown to inhibit oxidation of LDL cholesterol, according to a study in the *Annals of the New York Academy of Sciences*. Many scientists now believe that it is not only the amount of "bad" cholesterol in the blood that clogs our arteries but also the oxidation of it, causing the fatlike material to become rancid. Therefore, it is believed the soybean is capable of not only reducing cholesterol levels, but of preventing oxidative damage to LDL cholesterol as well.

PREVENTING STROKES

Takemichi Kanazawa and his colleagues at Hirosaki University School of Medicine in Japan studied the effects of soy creme in the blood of patients who had a stroke and in that of healthy persons. The soy creme suppressed the oxygen damage to proteins in their bodies and lowered cholesterol. Thus the Japanese researchers concluded that soy may be useful in the prevention and/or treatment of atherosclerosis, which can lead to blockage of the arteries to and in the brain, causing what we call a stroke and doctors call a "cerebral vascular accident."

MAGNIFICENT MAGNESIUM

Magnesium is a silver white, light metal that is high in some soybean products. A cup of EdenSoy brand soy milk, for example, contains 14 percent of the recommended daily intake of magnesium. Magnesium is needed for healthy arteries, bones, heart, muscles, nerves, and teeth. It activates enzymes needed to release energy. In 1992, it was reported in the British medical journal *Lancet* that injections of magnesium at the time of a heart attack reduced deaths by a fourth in a study of more than 2300 patients. The recommended daily intake of magnesium, according to the National Academy of Sciences, is forty milligrams for infants, 100 to 300 milligrams for children, and 350 milligrams for adults.

SOY AND THE MEDITERRANEAN DIET

Linoleic and linolenic acids are essential fatty acids. They cannot be manufactured in the human body and must be obtained from plants and that is why they are called "essential." They are both made from oleic acid in plants. Once ingested, these essential fatty acids are used to manufacture other potent substances. Linoleic acid is the most common dietary essential (for nutrition) fatty acid. It is required for growth. Soybean oil contains a good deal of linoleic acid.

It has been noted among researchers for many years that the French, who eat a high-fat diet, and the Italians have fewer heart attacks than Americans. Some say it is the wine they drink with their meals and others say it is the presence of alpha-linolenic acid (ALA) found in olive and canola oils. The typical Mediterranean diet has more bread, root vegetables, green vegetables, and fish, and less meat than the typical American diet. The Mediterraneans also eat a great deal of fruit.

In a French study of post–heart attack patients, one group of 302 patients was prescribed a diet of less saturated fats but more ALA. A control group of 302 patients ate their normal diets. After five years, the group that had the increased alpha-linolenic acid suffered only three deaths while the control group had sixteen deaths.

Gamma-linolenic acid (GLA), on the other hand, is derived from linoleic acid in the body during metabolic processing. GLA is similar, of course, to the heart-healthy ALA in the Mediterranean diet and to eicosapentaenoic acid (EPA), found in fish oil. Both GLA and EPA are basic building materials for prostaglandins, which work in our bodies very much like hormones. The prostaglandins created from GLA have been identified as contributing to the widening of blood vessels. They have also been found to help keep blood platelets from sticking together and causing clots that can produce heart attacks, strokes, and other vascular problems. GLA-constructed prostaglandins are also credited with helping to inhibit cholesterol production. As if that weren't enough, they are also said to improve circulation and strengthen the immune system.

In order to be converted to a beneficial hormonelike prostaglandin, linoleic acid in soy and other vegetables must first be processed into GLA by enzymes, the workhorses of the body. The conjecture is that many aspects of our lifestyles may reduce the ability of the enzymes to convert linoleic acid to GLA. These include high-fat diets, stress, and alcohol abuse. Aging, diabetes, and premenstrual syndrome may also have an effect. Theoretically, a boost of linoleic acid–containing soy in the diet may help GLA bypass the negative effects of the life style–produced enzyme blockers and thus enhance the formation of positively protective prostaglandins.

FOAM TO WASH OUT CHOLESTEROL?

Saponins are natural glycosides—compounds derived from sugars—that occur in many plants and are not associated with proteins of animal origin. Characterized by their ability to foam in water, saponins are used chiefly as foaming and emulsifying agents and detergents in household products. Saponins, however, also have the ability to liberate hemoglobin, which carries oxygen to the lungs, from red blood cells. Saponins have also been found to have an anti-inflammatory action similar to that of cortisone. Herbs that contain saponins, including goldenrod, chickweed, and wild yam, have long been used by folk medicine practitioners to soothe inflammation.

Saponins are thought to lower cholesterol either by blocking cholesterol absorption or by causing more cholesterol to be excreted from the body.

Robert Anderson and Walter Wolf of the Agricultural Research Service, U.S. Department of Agriculture, say that with the exception of alcohol-extracted concentrates, the saponins tend to remain with the protein products derived from soybeans. Fermentation, as in the preparation of miso, results in some degradation of the saponins and thus a lower saponin content compared with soybeans. The saponin content of soy products such as soy milk (see page 89), yuba (see page 91), tofu (see page 84), and natto (see page 97) ranges from 0.3 to 0.4 percent, about the same as soybeans. Cooked soybeans tend to be somewhat lower in saponin content, at 0.1 to 0.3 percent.

CHOLESTEROL COMPETITORS—PHYTOSTEROLS

Phytosterols are plant fatty alcohols that have a low toxicity. Most animal and human studies show that phytosterols reduce blood levels of cholesterol. Phytosterols are structurally very similar to cholesterol. As with the plant estrogens (see pages 38–40), phytosterols are believed to compete with cholesterol for absorption by the intestines, resulting in a drop in the cholesterol levels in the blood. Studies done in the 1970s reported that phytosterols lower cholesterol by as much as 40 percent. Drs. W. H. Long and P. J. Jones of McGill University in Canada reviewed eighty studies of dietary phytosterols in 1995. They concluded that phytosterols produce a wide range of therapeutic effects including not only cholesterol lowering but antitumor. They maintain that phytosterols should be studied further to maximize their usefulness as nonpharmacological substances to reduce atherosclerosis in the population.

A phytosterol, sitostanol, which is contained in soybeans, has been shown in an experimental margarine to lower serum cholesterol and LDL cholesterol. In the *New England Journal of Medicine,* November 16, 1995, T. A. Miettinen and colleagues reported that of 153 randomly selected subjects with mildly high cholesterol, 50 consumed margarine without sitostanol ester (the control group) and 102 consumed margarine containing up to 2.6 grams of sitostanol per day. The result was, after a year, cholesterol was 10.2 percent lower in the sitostanol group compared with an increase of 0.1 percent in the control group. The reduction in LDL in the sitostanol group was 14.1 percent and in the control group, 1.1 percent.

IS IT THYROID HORMONE?

Exactly how soybeans lower cholesterol is not known. William Forsythe III of the school of home economics at the University of Southern Mississippi in Hattiesburg is investigating whether it might be the bean's ability to stimulate the release of the thyroid hormone thyroxine. Thyroxine is produced by the butterfly-shaped thyroid gland located in the neck with a wing on either side of the windpipe. Thyroxine controls the rate of chemical reactions in the body. Generally, the more thyroxine, the faster the body works. The basic premise is that feeding soy protein lowers cholesterol concentration in the blood by causing an increase in blood thyroxine concentration. It is known that when thyroxine is elevated, cholesterol goes down.

AMINO ACID AT WORK?

When you eat a meal of soybeans or any other protein-containing food, digestive enzymes in your stomach and small intestines break apart the protein molecules into both "free" amino acids and small bunches of amino acids, called *peptides,* which are strung together head to tail. Your liver then controls the distribution of amino acids in your blood. As the amino acids move through your bloodstream, your body selects the particular amino acid building blocks it needs for its organs and their function.

Amino acids are extremely powerful in small doses and are versatile in changing roles, depending on where they are used in the body. That they are essential to your brain and body and are derived from foods, however, does not mean amino acids are harmless and should be taken lightly. The amino acid levels in your body are exquisitely balanced. By overloading your system with one, you can affect the levels of others, which may produce serious adverse effects on your body and brain.

Although scientists do not know how soy protein lowers cholesterol, one theory is that the amino acids in soy decrease the amount of insulin in the blood. When insulin levels are low, the liver manufactures less cholesterol. Wahida Karmally, director of nutrition at the Irving Center for Clinical Research at New York's Columbia-Presbyterian Medical Center, says that the protein in soybeans, with all of the essential amino acids, is very high quality for the plant world, low in saturated fat and without cholesterol.

ESSENTIAL AMINO ACID COMPOSITION OF THE SOYBEAN AND ESTIMATED DAILY REQUIREMENTS

AMINO ACID	SOYBEAN	ADULT	INFANT	CHILD
Cystine	1.2	13	58	27
Lysine	6.6	12	103	60
Leucine	7.6	14	161	45
Isoleucine	5.8	10	70	30
Methionine	1.1	13	58	27
Phenylalanine	4.8	14	125	27
Threonine	3.9	7	87	35
Tryptophan	1.2	3.5	17	4
Valine	5.2	10	93	33
Tyrosine	3.2	14	125	27

Soy protein causes less of a buildup of cholesterol than animal proteins because of the presence of arginine. Arginine is a nonessential, strongly alkaline amino acid that plays an important role in the production of urea excretion. Urea is a product of protein metabolism and is passed in the urine. It has been used for the treatment of liver disease. Cholesterol, of course, is made in the liver and therefore some researchers believe soybean arginine may well play some part in counteracting the high cholesterol effect of other amino acids in our bodies.

COULD IT BE THE B's?

Homocysteine levels in the blood have recently been reported to be as important or even more important than cholesterol levels in contributing to clogging of the arteries. Homocysteine helps the body to process the amino acid methionine. Alberto Ascherio and Walter Willett of the departments of epidemiology and nutrition at Harvard School of Public Health pointed out at The First International Symposium on the Role of Soy in Preventing and Treating Chronic Disease held in Mesa, Arizona, in 1994, that increased blood homocysteine levels may be caused by inadequate intakes of vitamin B_6, folate, or vitamin B_{12}, which are cofactors in converting homocysteine to methionine, or by high intakes of methionine.

The level of methionine is very low in soybeans, while the B vitamins, including folate, B_6, niacin, thiamine, riboflavin, and pantothenic acid, are abundant. There is a theory that the low levels of methionine in soybeans may be beneficial to the heart and blood vessels (see page 25).

IS IT THE FLAVONOIDS?

Flavonoids are a large group of compounds widely distributed throughout nature. Soybeans contain flavonoid compounds called *isoflavones,* which are plant estrogens. They are weaker than human hormones but they aim for the same receptors on human cells and are believed to be able to block human estrogens—a sort of "I got here first and you can't play."

Estrogen has been widely credited with protecting young women against cardiovascular disease, and estrogen replacement in menopausal women has been widely reported to reduce their risk of heart disease.

Elaine Raines and Russell Ross of the Department of Pathology at the University of Washington in Seattle maintained at the Arizona symposium on soybeans and health that they have another theory. They are testing whether increased levels of isoflavonoids, in particular genistein—which is unique to soybeans—inhibit cell stickiness, alter growth factor activity, and inhibit cell proliferation involved in hardening and clogging of the arteries. These compounds have antioxidant properties that may be playing a direct role in soy's beneficial effects on the heart and blood vessels.

Josiah Wilcox and Barbara Blumenthal of the Division of Hematology and Oncology at Emory University Medical School said at the same symposium they found that generally injuries that remove or disrupt the endothelial cells lining blood vessels stimulate formation of blood vessel lesions. One of the first events after such cell lining injury is the generation of thrombin at the site of injury. Thrombin is an enzyme in the blood that helps it clot. The clot formation leads to artery-clogging hard, fatty bumps (atherosclerotic plaques), which grow for many years. Genistein, the isoflavonoid derived from soy products, has been shown to inhibit thrombin formation. The Emory researchers therefore believe genistein may affect the progression of hardening and clogging of the arteries and blood vessels.

Anderson and Wolf of the Agricultural Research Service say that processing generally does not remove the

isoflavones from soybean protein products except for concentrates prepared by alcohol extraction. Lowering of the
isoflavone contents of some soybean foods may also result
from dilution by the addition of other ingredients, such as
salt in miso.

Susan Potter, principal investigator in the soy-
cholesterol studies at the University of Illinois, is incorporating soy protein into baked foods, drinks, soups, and
entrées during six-month feeding trials with about seventy-
five postmenopausal women who have high blood fats. Researchers are looking at the effects of soy protein and soy
isoflavones to evaluate the risk of cardiovascular disease
and bone density in relation to osteoporosis. Preliminary
findings are encouraging, Potter said. In fact, soy protein
apparently lowered the women's blood cholesterol by 10
to 25 percent.

THE BEAN AND OBESITY

A major risk factor in heart disease is obesity. Many of us
are overweight. It is estimated that 46.3 million American
adults are more than 20 percent over their desirable
weight. Obesity exists in 24.4 percent of white males, 24.7
percent of black males, 25.1 percent of white females, and
43.8 percent of black females. Extra pounds make the
heart work harder. Just think how you feel when you carry
a heavy package upstairs. Being overweight not only
makes your heart pump harder, it can also raise blood pressure, constrict your lungs, and make your body require
more oxygen.

It is not easy to lose weight, as we all well know, but
substituting soy products for some fat-laden, high-calorie
meat and dairy products can certainly help.

HIGH BLOOD PRESSURE AND THE BEAN

It is estimated that nearly 60 million Americans have high blood pressure. Physicians generally diagnose high blood pressure when an otherwise healthy adult has consistent readings above 140/90. The upper number in a blood pressure reading, called the systolic pressure, is a measurement made when the heart is contracting. The lower number in a blood pressure reading, called the diastolic pressure, is recorded when the heart is at rest.

Elevated blood pressure means the heart is working harder than normal, putting both the heart and the arteries under great strain. This may contribute to heart attacks, strokes, kidney failure, and atherosclerosis. When the heart is forced to work harder than normal for an extended time, it tends to enlarge. A slightly enlarged heart may function well, but one that is significantly enlarged has a hard time adequately meeting the demands put upon it.

Arteries and blood vessels also suffer the effect of high blood pressure. Over time, they become scarred, hardened, and less elastic. This may occur as we age, but elevated blood pressure speeds the process and is believed to accelerate atherosclerosis.

In almost all cases the cause of high blood pressure is unknown. In a few instances, the high blood pressure is due to an underlying problem such as kidney disease, tumor of the adrenal gland, or a defect of the aorta, the largest artery emanating from the heart.

Since high blood pressure usually presents no symptoms, many people don't know they have it or if they do know, they stop taking medication prescribed for it. Uncontrolled high blood pressure can lead not only to heart problems but also to strokes and kidney failure. This is why it is called the "silent killer."

Medications are prescribed when blood pressure cannot be lowered by losing weight, reducing salt intake, and increasing exercise.

Soybeans have been found to help lower blood pressure. The theory is that something in soybeans may act like a type of drug that is widely prescribed today for high blood pressure—angiotensin-converting enzyme (ACE) inhibitors. These drugs act on the body's production of angiotensin, an enzyme that causes arteries to constrict. ACE-inhibiting enzyme has been isolated from soy sauce by Japanese researchers. In the laboratory, the soy ACE inhibitor reduced blood pressure in hypertensive rats. Soy sauce in its entirety, of course, contains a lot of salt that can raise blood pressure in sensitive people. It is possible, however, that whatever it is in the sauces or other soy products will be isolated and become a *nutraceutical* for high blood pressure in humans.

COULD IT BE JUST AVOIDING MEAT AND DAIRY PRODUCTS?

Many soy skeptics say that you will derive cholesterol-lowering benefits just by substituting any vegetarian dishes for meat and dairy dishes.

Dr. Erdman of the University of Illinois points out that participants in their soy studies were all on the American Heart Association's recommended diet, which is low in animal and dairy fat. The only dietary difference between the controls and the ones who received the soy protein *was the soy protein*.

Ronald Krauss, M.D., chairman of the American Heart Association's Nutrition Committee and senior scientist at the University of California at Berkeley, issued the following statement after the August 3, 1995, *New En-*

gland Journal of Medicine article on soy's capacity to lower cholesterol received such media attention:

> The use of soy protein in moderation is entirely consistent with the American Heart Association dietary guidelines. Based on much stronger and more extensive evidence than the meta-analysis report (in the *New England Journal* article, August 3, 1995), these recommendations call for limiting sources of animal fat, which is associated with animal protein, and consuming more vegetables and fruits. It is, of course, quite reasonable to choose soy-based food products within an overall balanced diet.
>
> However, as with other published studies of specific foods, the AHA is concerned about the potential for some people to focus on one narrow and not fully established dietary approach and perhaps deflect attention from broader-based dietary principles. It is not clear how a soy effect, which is rather modest when consumed in practical amounts, matches up against the effects of other cholesterol-lowering dietary changes. We also need to have more studies aimed at understanding the mechanisms of the presumed soy effect. For example, if, as suggested, plant estrogen content of soy protein is of importance, overall biologic impact, including conceivable risks with high intakes, needs to be better understood.
>
> The conclusion of the 1993 American Heart Association Rationale of the Diet-Heart Statement stands that animal work on

soy protein is solid while effects in humans, with a few exceptions, are not nearly so convincing. No single report can be conclusive, and most studies used in the meta-analysis did not show significant LDL reduction. Meta-analysis may give scientists more confidence that there is an effect, but we cannot use this averaged information to make specific dietary recommendations for the public. The AHA's Nutrition Committee is looking more closely at recent data and can be expected to develop more specific guidelines as research information accumulates.

SUMMING IT UP

Soy cuts cholesterol about as much as low-fat diets do, according to Margaret Cook-Newell, a coauthor of the Kentucky meta-analysis study of soy reported in the *New England Journal of Medicine*. Cook-Newell said the American Heart Association's diet can reduce cholesterol by 5 to 10 percent; a very low-fat, high-fiber diet can reduce levels 13 to 19 percent; and drugs can lower levels 10 to 20 percent.

There are no side effects from soy except for the few who are sensitive to it, but Cook-Newell, a dietitian and doctoral student in nutrition at the University of Kentucky, warns that regarding soy foods as a quick health fix is the wrong approach.

She and her colleagues encourage Americans to begin by converting a quarter of the average 100 grams of protein they eat each day (mostly from meat and dairy products) to soy foods.

You do need to eat more than a chunk of tofu to get

the effects. In the studies James Anderson and his colleagues analyzed, subjects received an average of forty-seven grams of soy protein a day—about half the protein consumed in the average American diet. A half-cup of tofu contains eight to thirteen grams of protein. That could mean three or more servings of soy foods every day. But even twenty-five grams (⅛ cup) of soy protein daily can lower cholesterol 2 to 3 percent, the researchers say.

"We're not telling people to add this soy protein to a high-fat, high-calorie diet, because it's not going to give you the effect," Cook-Newell says. "We advocate a well-balanced diet. Just make a gradual change."

Is the key factor in protecting the heart and blood vessels soy protein or any other substances mentioned in this chapter? Do the beneficial effects require that all be present? Could it be, as some skeptics say, that just substituting a vegetable protein for meat and dairy protein produces the benefits? The proof will ultimately be in the bean!

Chapter 2

How Soy Protects
Against Cancer

Can as little as 1 cup of soy milk, 1 cup tofu, or ¼ cup soy powder per day lower your risk of cancer?

Epidemiologists are citing the low rates of certain cancers in the Orient where soy foods are consumed in large quantities and reports are flooding the scientific literature about the potential anticancer benefits of soy. For example:

- In the United States, it has been reported that women consuming soy foods had 50 percent less incidence of cancer than those who did not eat soy-based products.
- Breast cancer and prostate cancer are much lower in the Far East where people eat twenty to fifty times more soy products than Americans.
- Bean curd has been noted to have a protective effect on stomach cancer risk among Japanese-Hawaiians and lung cancer among Chinese miners.
- Soy products appear to protect premenopausal women from breast cancer in Singapore.

What is it in the tiny soybean that might account for its anticancer properties?

Scientists now believe its chemopreventive benefits are probably due to its *nonnutritional* substances once thought to be unimportant or even damaging to human health.

Drs. David Alberts and Dava Garcia of the Department of Medicine at the University of Arizona in Tucson pointed out at The First International Symposium on the Role of Soy in Preventing and Treating Chronic Disease held in Arizona in February 1994 that chemoprevention is an area of cancer research with perhaps the greatest potential for reducing cancer death rates.

"Despite increased funding for cancer research afforded by the passage of the National Cancer Act of 1971 and a multitude of treatment advances over the past thirty years, cancer death rates have continued to rise," they said.

Cancer is now believed to be a two-stage process with *initiation*—exposure to a cancer-causing substance—and *promotion*—stimulation by another substance that makes the first become active. It had been assumed once cells have been both *initiated* and *promoted* they inevitably go haywire and become cancerous.

The aim of cancer chemoprevention, however, the two Arizona researchers and many other scientists maintain, is to circumvent this process through the use of nontoxic nutrients or drugs. Because the time span between tumor *initiation* and frank malignancy often exceeds a decade, there is considerable time to prevent promotion and to halt or reverse cancer development.

PROTEASE INHIBITORS

Among the weapons to stop cancer development, according to a number of prominent researchers, are the nonnutritive substances in soybeans called *protease inhibitors*. They are found in the reproductive parts of soybeans and other beans, rice, and potatoes. Protease inhibitors are believed to provide these edibles with natural protection to prevent seed digestion by insects, thus assuring survival of the plant species.

Because they block the activity of an enzyme that aids the digestion of proteins, protease inhibitors were once thought to interfere with nutrition. Walter Troll, Ph.D., of New York University Medical Center, who is conducting cancer studies with protease inhibitors, notes that the U.S. Department of Agriculture spent a lot of time removing protease inhibitors from soybeans because it was believed their removal would make young children grow better.

Ann Kennedy, Ph.D., when at the Harvard School of Public Health's Department of Cancer Biology in Boston, and her colleagues there found that protease inhibitors may be capable of neutralizing the effect of a wide range of cancer-causing agents, from radiation and hormones to potent components of diesel exhaust.

What Dr. Kennedy and her coworkers reported was that even brief exposure of *initiated* and/or *promoted* cells to minute quantities of certain protease inhibitors—such as the Bowman-Birk Inhibitor (BBI) derived from soybeans—not only prevents the transformation of those cells into cancers, but also "reprograms" their precancerous changes back to the pre-initiation normal state. Dr. Kennedy and her group reported treatment with the protease inhibitor from soybeans could start 45 to 135 days after the beginning of exposure to a cancer-causing agent and still suppress the malignant process. The only real limit to the achievement seems to be the dose of the cancer-causing *initiator*. If the amount of cancer-causing agent is too high, the protease inhibitor may reduce but not stop tumor development.

Dr. Kennedy says some cancer researchers have labeled her findings "heresy" on the assumption that changes during cancer *initiation* were irreversible. Her research suggests that both *initiating* and *promoting* changes are indeed reversible with protease inhibitors.

Dr. Kennedy, who is now at the Department of Radiation Oncology at the University of Pennsylvania, presented a paper on BBI and soy at The First International Conference on the Role of Soy in Preventing and Treating Chronic Disease held in Arizona in 1994. She said the Bowman-Birk Inhibitor is the compound in soybeans that has shown the greatest suppression of cancer development in animals.

She said she and her colleagues have observed that BBI can completely prevent colon cancer and suppress liver cancer by 71 percent, cancer in the lining of the mouth by 86 percent, and cancer in the lungs by 48 percent.

To understand how BBI and other nonnutritive substances in soybeans work, both Drs. Kennedy and Troll are focusing on the protease inhibitors' recently identified ability to restrain the action of cancer-causing genes (oncogenes) carried by viruses. It is generally assumed that specific cancer-causing genes must be "turned on" for cancer to develop and the hope is that protease inhibitors will keep those bad genes from becoming active.

The new class of AIDS drugs causing a great deal of hope, such as Merck's Crixivan, are, in fact, *protease* inhibitors!

TRYPSIN INHIBITORS

Other protease inhibitors receiving scientific attention are the trypsin inhibitors located in the part that stores nutrition for the soybean itself. Trypsin is an enzyme that helps us digest proteins.

Trypsin inhibitors display anticarcinogenic properties, according to Robert L. Anderson and Walter J. Wolf of the Agricultural Research Service, U.S. Department of Agriculture, at The First International Symposium on the Role of Soy in Preventing and Treating Chronic Disease held in Mesa, Arizona, in 1994. Trypsin inhibitors are protein and subject to inactivation by heat. A fully toasted soy flour will have a trypsin inhibitor level of only eight to nine milligrams per gram of flour while raw defatted flour may have twenty-eight to thirty-two milligrams per gram. Oriental and other soybean foods are generally low in trypsin inhibitor. Tofu, which is made from heated soybean milk, has a trypsin inhibitor content of about nine milligrams per gram of protein. Soy infant formula made from soy protein isolate with the addition of other nutrients has only 0.3 to three milligrams per gram.

PLANT ESTROGENS

Isoflavones—plant estrogens—were also long considered antinutritional, but, like protease inhibitors, they are now of great interest because of their newly recognized anti-cancer activities. It has been known since 1931 that soybeans contain high amounts—up to 100 to 300 milligrams per 100 grams—of two major isoflavones, genistein and daidzein. A third one, glycetein, was discovered forty years later. Still another estrogen, equol, is similar to the powerful human estrogen, estradiol-17. Equol was found by Dr. Adlercreutz and his colleagues at the University of Helsinki to be lower in women with breast cancer than women without the disease.

Scientists from several countries, on the other hand, have found much higher levels of the estrogen genistein in the urine of people who eat a traditional Japanese diet than in those who eat the typical Western diet. Genistein is a powerful anticarcinogen in test tubes where it directly inhibits the growth of a wide range of cancer cells. In the laboratory, Dr. Lothar Schweigerer and his colleagues at Heidelberg University, for example, discovered that genistein blocks an event called angiogenesis, the growth of new blood vessels that nourish malignant tumors. Once a tumor grows beyond a millimeter, it must foster the growth of new blood vessels around it. When it is fully vascularized, the malignancy then receives the oxygen and nourishment it needs to grow and eventually sends fatal metastatic colonies elsewhere. By inhibiting blood vessel growth, genistein may keep new tumors from growing beyond harmless dimensions. That could have implications for the treatment of solid tumors, including malignancies of the breast, prostate, and brain.

Another reason why soy estrogens such as genistein may help prevent breast cancers may lie in competitive blocking of the kind of estrogens produced in women's bodies. Both plant and human estrogens appear to dock at the same receptor sites on human cells. Animal-derived estrogens stimulate tissues, while plant-derived estrogens are quite inert. Breasts have been found to contain more of the self-produced estrogen than does surrounding noncancerous breast tissue. The plant form of estrogen has been found to be elevated in women who are vigorous athletes and in those who eat soy and, to a lesser extent, cruciferous vegetables such as broccoli and kale.

Under grants from the National Institutes of Health, genistein is now being tested in patients who have breast cancer, prostate cancer, melanomas (a potentially deadly skin cancer), leukemia, and Kaposi's sarcoma, a cancer frequently linked to AIDS.

Soy foods that are rich in genistein include whole

soybeans, tofu, soy milk, and tempeh. No other commonly consumed foods contain it.

Although the study of anticancer phytoestrogens is science in progress, if the effects are due to the isoflavones, this places particular emphasis on soy because the iso-flavones have a very limited distribution in nature. Stephen Holt, M.D., president of Natus, Inc., has developed Genista, a soy protein isolate with isoflavones (see Where to Get More Information, page 171). This product is probably the forerunner of many "health" products made from soy.

Plant lignans are other phytoestrogens. They occur widely and are obtained from roots, heartwood, foliage, fruit, and resins of plants. The lignans enterolactone and enterodiol occur in humans and animals. They have been reported to possess anticancer, antiviral, bactericidal, and fungistatic properties. The lignans are normal constituents of human urine, blood plasma, and feces. They are higher in the blood of vegetarians than meat eaters.

POLYPHENOLS

Polyphenols are compounds found in many plants including soybeans, garlic, green tea, cereal grains, cruciferous vegetables such as broccoli, umbelliferous vegetables such as celery, citrus fruits, solanaceous vegetables such as potatoes, and curcuma such as ginger, licorice root, and flaxseed. Polyphenols are believed to act at both the *initiation* and *promotion* stages of cancer development. They have been reported to interfere with tumor promotion by dampening hormones as described above for plant estrogens. Polyphenols act as "garbage collectors," disposing of cell-damaging mutagens and cancer-causing agents. Phenols are used as disinfectants and anesthetics for the skin.

TERPENES—ANTIOXIDANTS

Terpenes are in a class of organic compounds containing only carbon and hydrogen and occur in most essential oils and plant resins. They are found in soybeans as well as garlic, cereal grains, many vegetables, citrus fruits, and licorice root. Among terpene derivatives are camphor and menthol. Terpenes act as antioxidants and are believed to interrupt both *initiation* by cancer-causing agents and *promotion* by hormones. It is yet to be determined how much they contribute to the soybean's apparent anticancer effects but it is known that antioxidants inhibit cell damage from oxygen. Most of the damaging effects of oxygen results from free radicals. Free radicals are highly reactive molecules generated when a cell "burns" its food with oxygen to fuel life processes. Free radicals act like "loose cannons," rolling around and damaging cells. This damage is thought to be a first step in cancer development. It has been shown that antioxidants such as vitamin C, vitamin E, and a number of phytochemicals found in fruits, vegetables, and legumes such as soybeans can suppress free radical cell damage.

FIGHTING PHYTATES

Soybeans are high in phytates, the plant storage form of the mineral phosphorus, which is necessary for every tissue in the body. Phytates are chelates—they bind with and carry out from the intestines minerals such as calcium and iron. At one time, these antinutrients were in such disfavor that agriculturists tried to grow soybeans with low levels of phytates. Researchers now believe that they may have been wrong. For example, in a review of fifty-nine studies in

1993, Drs. E. Graf and J. W. Eaton suggested that it is not only the fiber in the diet that may protect us from breast and colon cancer but the phytates, which are high in high-fiber foods.

MAYBE IT'S DUE TO LOW-COUNT AMINO ACID

The cancer-preventing effects of soybeans have been attributed to the presence of antinutrients such as the phyto-estrogens genistein and daidzein, protease inhibitors, and the phytates, as you have read in this chapter. An important anticancer property of soybean may be not what is in them but what is missing—a high level of the essential amino acid methionine. In a paper presented at the 1994 international symposium on soy in Arizona, E. J. Hawrylewicz and colleagues at the Department of Research of Mercy Hospital in Chicago said that the metastatic growth in the lungs of a tumor was inhibited in animals by feeding a soy protein. The development of mammary (breast) tumors induced by cancer-causing agents was inhibited during the *promotional* phase in rats fed soy protein. The effect was reversed when methionine was added to their diet. Rats fed a soybean protein diet supplement with methionine developed 1.4 times the total number of mammary tumors than either the unsupplemented soybean- or casein-fed rats after exposure to a cancer-causing agent. Casein is the major protein in cows' milk. Additional studies demonstrated that after surgical removal of a mammary tumor, growth of additional tumors was inhibited when the diet was changed from casein to soy protein. The concentration of the essential amino acid methionine in soybean protein is significantly less than found in milk protein, and a deficiency in methionine may prove to be one of the elements in soy that puts a damper on tumor proliferation.

SAPONINS

Saponins are compounds derived from sugars and are found in many plants. They are the main protein supplier in many vegetarian diets and are not associated with proteins of animal origin. There are at least five saponins in soybeans that provide one of the most important sources of these dietary substances.

Exactly how saponins fight cancer is not known but it is believed it has something to do with their action on the cell membrane since saponins are not absorbed into the cell.

Although research with soy saponins is in its early stages, it is hoped that they will prove to be useful in protecting the lining of the intestines from cancer-causing agents.

The saponin content of several oriental foods such as soy milk, yuba, tofu, and natto is in the 0.3 to 0.4 range, about the same as uncooked and unprocessed soybeans. Miso and cooked soybeans tend to have a somewhat lower saponin content.

INOSITOL—THE CANCER-FIGHTING PHYTIC ACID

First identified in 1855, inositol hexaphosphate is a member of the vitamin B family and is widely found in the plant kingdom in small amounts. It regulates vital cellular functions in mammals. According to Abulkalam Shamsuddin, Ph.D., of the Department of Pathology at the University of Maryland, who spoke at The First International Symposium on Soy in Arizona, inositol has "striking anticancer potential—preventive as well as therapeutic" both in the test tube and in living animals.

In addition to reducing cell proliferation, it often results in turning malignant cells back to normal, Dr. Shamsuddin said.

Because inositol hexaphosphate is abundant in high-fiber diets, the studies at the University of Maryland may explain, at least in part, the epidemiologic observation that high-fiber diets are associated with a lower incidence of certain cancers.

WHICH SOY PRODUCTS HAVE THE MOST ANTICANCER POTENTIAL?

Soy flour, which is made by defatting dehulled flakes and grinding, has an isoflavone profile approximately that of soybeans and so do textured vegetable protein (TVP) products.

Shoyu, Japanese-style soy sauce, is produced through a complex microbial fermentation of soy. During its manufacture, characteristic flavors and aromas develop due to the action of microbes and reactions between various chemical substances.

As far back as 1980, Dr. Michael Pariza reported at the American Chemical Society meeting in Dallas, Texas, that shoyu contains an unidentified antitumor substance. Dr. Pariza, who is a director of the Food Research Institute at the University of Wisconsin, noted that mice fed benzopyrene, a potent cancer-causing agent, developed fewer stomach tumors when they were fed soy sauce than when they were not.

Dr. Pariza and his associates at the University of Wisconsin's Department of Food Microbiology and Toxicology wanted to know why Japanese-style soy sauce inhibited cancer of the stomach in animals. They extracted a major flavor/aroma compound from soy sauce, HEMF [4-hydroxy-2(or 5)-ethyl-5(or 2)-methyl-3(2H)furanone], and found it to be an antioxidant as well as a powerful anticancer agent. The Wisconsin researchers discovered that in animals, HEMF inhibited tumor *promotion*. HEMF is also found in tofu and other researchers are interested in its anticancer potential.

Tofu, a soybean-based food that has become increasingly popular in the United States, contains high levels of the plant estrogen daidzein, which is also believed to be an anticancer chemical. Tofu is greatly reduced in isoflavones because of the water processing used during its manufacture. Tempeh is even lower in isoflavone content than tofu. Until recently, therefore, scientists did not believe that such soy products contained enough phytoestrogens to fight cancer. Johanna Dwyer, Ph.D., professor of nutrition at Tufts University and her colleagues found out, however, that different brands of tofu contain from seventy-three to ninety-seven micrograms of the phytoestrogen daidzein per gram of tofu. They wrote in *The Journal of the American Dietetic Association* in 1994 that as tofu intake increases in the American diet, the daidzein may help prevent breast cancer. Tofu, they noted, also contains other anticancer chemicals such as the phytoestrogen genestein and HEMF, which may help explain why the Japanese who use a lot of soy products have far less breast and prostate cancer than Americans.

As you have read, many researchers believe it is the plant estrogens—the isoflavonoids—that may be a large factor in dietary cancer prevention. Which soy products contain the most palatable isoflavonoids and how much of the substances do you have to eat to obtain the cancer-protective benefit?

Andrea Hutchins, Joanne Slavin, and Johanna

Lampe of the Department of Food Science and Human Ecology of the University of Minnesota compared the effects of soybean fermentation on isoflavonoid excretion. In the May 1995 issue of *The Journal of the American Dietetic Association,* they reported on their study, which involved seventeen healthy men between the ages of twenty and forty recruited from the University of Minnesota Twin Cities community. The men were screened to exclude those who had gastrointestinal disorders, food allergies, alcohol intake greater than two drinks a day, smoked, had taken antibiotics within the past six months, regularly used prescription or nonprescription medications, or had dietary habits that were not representative of the general population. The participants' test diets included soybean pieces, tempeh, or tomato-based soy mixtures. The Minnesota researchers found that the subjects' urinary content of isoflavonoids increased most with the consumption of tempeh compared with the other soybean products—an indication of the beneficial plant estrogen levels in the body.

The Minnesota researchers point out that several epidemiologic studies suggest that as little as one serving of soy each day—for example four ounces of tofu—can lower cancer risk. Some researchers estimate that isoflavonoid intake could be met by consuming four to twelve ounces of several soy products such as roasted soybeans, tempeh, tofu, or soy milk. In the Minnesota study, the men consumed 3.7 ounces of tempeh, which provided an average of 0.5 milligrams isoflavone per kilogram of body weight per day.

Andrea Hutchins and her University of Minnesota colleagues maintain that although the level of soy consumption believed to be necessary for a reduction in cancer risk is currently above the average American soy intake of three grams per day, the ingestion of soy products by Americans increased approximately 40 percent between

1980 and 1990. Hutchins says that with the continuation of this trend and the addition of new soy products to the market, many Americans could reach these proposed levels of soy consumption in the near future.

Purdue University researchers in Indiana, in addition, are exploring the possibility of developing a new type of soybean to produce proteins used in cancer therapy for humans and animals. Laboratory cultures now used to make those potentially therapeutic proteins are difficult to produce, but growing the proteins in soybean fields could lower the cost of these anticancer nutraceuticals for consumers.

POTENTIAL ADVERSE EFFECTS OF SOYBEANS

As with any beneficial medication, there are side effects and dosage restrictions. Irvin Liener, Ph.D., of the Department of Biochemistry at the University of Minnesota pointed out at the Arizona meeting on soybeans and health in 1994 that the prolonged feeding of raw soy flour to rats results in the development of overgrowth and tumors of the pancreas, including malignancies. Dr. Mark Messina, who was formerly with the National Cancer Institute, said that only raw soybeans showed this effect in rats, so don't eat raw soybeans.

There is also the question about how much protease inhibitors in soybeans may affect protein nutrition. Dr. Liener says that it should be emphasized that all of these adverse effects are seen when protease inhibitors are present in relatively high concentrations in the diet and may be completely unrelated to the anticarcinogenic effects seen at low concentrations of the Bowman-Birk Inhibitor.

John C. Mirsalis, Ph.D., associate director of toxicology at SRI (formerly Stanford Research Institute), investigated the toxicology of soybean flakes in mice under a National Cancer Institute grant.

"There was some reporting of pancreatic problems in rats," he said in an interview with the author. "We were studying licorice root at the same time. Licorice root did cause a variety of problems in 25 percent of the mice, but soybean flakes did not."

Dr. John Erdman, Jr., of the University of Illinois, who is conducting studies on soybeans and cholesterol, said in an interview that there has been no evidence that soybeans or any soybean derivatives adversely affect the pancreas in humans.

Dr. Mirsalis, whose Ph.D. is in the field of genetics and toxicology, said that data in animals and in humans clearly show that soybeans are beneficial as a cancer chemopreventative agent.

"They clearly are beneficial, whether it is the protease inhibitors themselves or some other component, such as the flavones. We don't know for sure."

Dr. Mirsalis explained in the interview that one component of the detoxification pathway is *conjugation*. He said he believes something in the soybean binds with the carcinogen and causes the cancer-causing agent to be rapidly excreted in the urine.

Dr. Messina, a pioneer in soy cancer research, wrote in a review article in *Nutrition and Cancer* that of the twenty-six animal studies of experimental cancer-causing agents in which diets were employed containing soy or soybean isoflavones, 65 percent reported positive effects. No studies reported that soy intake increased tumor development. The epidemiologic data are also inconsistent. Protective effects were observed for both hormone- and nonhormone-related cancers. While a definitive statement that soy reduces cancer risks cannot be made at this time, Dr. Messina says there is sufficient evidence of a protective effect to warrant continued investigation.

Chapter 3

How Soy Helps to Ease Digestive Problems

The Finns have a high-fat diet and the Japanese have a low-fat diet. If colon cancer death rates in the United States were at the level of Finland, the number of Americans dying each year from colon cancer would drop from 60,000 to below 20,000. If the United States had the same breast cancer mortality rate as Japan, the number of American women dying each year from breast cancer would drop from 46,000 to 11,000, according to Peter Greenwald, M.D., director of the Division of Cancer Prevention and Control of the National Cancer Institute in Bethesda, Maryland.

What do the Finns and the Japanese have in common in their diets that most of us do not that may account for their lower cancer rate? Many researchers believe the answer is sufficient fiber!

The soybean, especially its outer hull, is one of the best sources of dietary fiber—six grams per one cup of cooked beans. When soybeans are processed into meal, protein products, and oil, the hull is removed. These hulls are then further processed to create a fiber additive for breads, cereals, and snacks.

How is the fiber in soybeans and other foods metabolized by our digestive system?

The large intestine is a tube about two inches in diameter and about five feet long. It consists of two main sections, the colon and the rectum. The small intestine opens into a pouchlike chamber called the cecum, which is the first part of the colon. The rest of the colon then runs up the right side of the abdomen, across the rib cage, and down the left side, thus forming a frame for the multi-looped small intestine. The rectum is a short tube about five inches long that leads downward from the end of the colon to the anus. Fluid and various mineral salts from the intestinal contents are absorbed into the bloodstream through the membranous wall of the colon, while indigestible solids are compacted and moved toward the rectum where waste is stored until it is released through the anus.

The large intestine may be vulnerable to many ailments for several reasons. It is particularly prone to infection-caused inflammation, and it is more susceptible than other sections of the digestive tract to tumors and polyps. Moreover, the large intestines can be adversely affected by many foods we eat. The evidence for this is in the disorders of the rectum and colon that are far more common in the United States than in Africa and Asia, where there is more fiber in the diet.

It takes about twelve to fourteen hours for contents to make the lap around the large intestines. The movement of food there is more unhurried than in the small intestine. Contractions move it along. Nerve reflexes signal the urge for a bowel movement. A final valve arrangement of two ringlike voluntary muscles, anal sphincters, terminates the digestive tract.

In contrast to the normally germ-free stomach, the colon is lavishly populated with bacteria, harmless, resident intestinal flora. A large part of the feces is composed of bacteria along with the stuff you have eaten as well as substances eliminated from the blood and shed from the intestinal walls.

One of the most common causes of lower abdominal pain is irritable colon syndrome. In this condition, the colon overreacts to various stimuli, such as emotions or certain foods. Symptoms may include cramping pain in the lower abdomen, bloating, passing of gas, distention, or a generalized abdominal ache.

Soy-based formulas are widely used for infants who cannot tolerate cow's milk. In a report in 1993 by Dr. K. H. Brown and colleagues at the University of California, Davis, thirty-four hospitalized male infants between two and twenty-four months, who were suffering from severe, watery diarrhea, were randomly assigned to receive a soy-protein isolate, lactose-free formula with added soy fiber. The addition of the soy fiber to the soy formula significantly and markedly reduced the duration of liquid stool excretion, the California researchers reported.

Constipation, on the other hand, is the difficult or infrequent passage of stools. Constipation may be a sign of obstruction of the colon caused by a tumor or a cancer. If you suffer chronically from it, you should consult a physician. The treatment, of course, lies in the cause, but it is well known that fiber helps to prevent or to ease constipation.

There are basically two types of fiber—insoluble and soluble—and soybeans have them both. Insoluble dietary fiber is believed to be mainly a bulking agent, increasing stool weight and decreasing transit time. Soluble fiber is associated with lowered cholesterol in the blood and improved blood sugar regulation in diabetics. There is still not complete understanding of how both types of fibers work. In the colon, some forms of dietary fiber are fermented by bacteria. Other forms resist this fermentation and pass unchanged from the body in the stool.

Soluble fibers are believed to benefit human health by binding to artery-clogging cholesterol and to potentially harmful hormones. Fiber's grabbing of cholesterol and hormones causes these substances to be eliminated from the body more quickly. These same fibers raise the acidity of the large intestine that prevents the recycling of potentially harmful bile acids that are one of the major byproducts of cholesterol metabolism and are believed to be involved in the development of colon cancer. Plant estrogens, which are also plentiful in soy foods, protect the colon from injury from bile acids.

Soluble fiber absorbs water and thus increases the water content and size of the stool. This may also, it is believed, reduce the concentration of chemicals that may cause irritation and/or cancer.

PROMOTING REGULARITY

Soybeans are legumes and legumes of all types are very helpful in promoting a healthy colon and bowel regularity. In fact, the fiber you eat has the following benefits:

- Stimulates saliva
- Dilutes contents of the stomach and prolongs storage
- Dilutes contents of the small intestine and delays absorption
- Dilutes contents of the large intestine and bacteria, traps water, and binds
- Softens and enlarges the stool and prevents straining

All the above may help ease or prevent diverticular disease and ulcerative colitis. In diverticulosis, there are little sacs (diverticula) in the walls of the intestines and gallbladder that become inflamed. In ulcerative colitis, there are sores and ulcers inside the colon usually accompanied by bloody diarrhea. One out of every twenty people who have ulcerative colitis eventually develops cancer of the colon.

Cancer of the large intestine is the third most common malignancy. Only lung cancer and breast cancer are more common in the United States. Colon cancer is the second leading cause of cancer deaths in the United States. Colon cancer will be diagnosed in 111,000 people this year and will cause about 51,000 deaths in the United States.

A combined analysis of thirteen international studies by Geoffrey Howe, Jr., M.D., of the University of Toronto and his colleagues provided strong evidence that high intakes of fiber-rich foods decrease cancer risk for both the colon and the rectum. They found that in twelve of thirteen studies, eating lots of fiber in foods can indeed slash the risk of colon cancer about in half.

Dr. Howe, writing in the *Journal of the National Cancer Institute of Canada* in 1994, maintained that a high-fiber, lower-fat diet may be especially important for persons at high risk of developing colorectal cancer, such as middle-aged and older adults and persons with a family history of the disease.

He and colleagues figure that if everyone ate about 70 percent more fiber than usual, the rates of colon and rectal cancers would drop 31 percent, preventing an annual 50,000 new cases in both men and women of all ages.

This would mean adding at least thirteen grams of food fiber daily for most people. There is about six grams of fiber per cup of cooked soybeans, eight grams of fiber in half a cup of green soybeans without the pods, one gram in four ounces of tofu, and 4.3 grams in 3½ ounces of defatted soy flour. Soy products, therefore, can not only lower our cholesterol and our risk of cancer, but they can also keep us regular.

Still, some cancer specialists are skeptical that fiber itself protects against colon cancer. They note that diets rich in animal fat may promote colon cancer and high-fiber diets may discourage colon cancer not because of the fiber but because such diets are generally low in fat content.

The National Cancer Institute currently does not promote the use of fiber supplements or fiber-fortified foods for the general public because the specific food components in fiber-rich foods that may protect against cancer have not yet been identified. Although dietary fiber supplements are not harmful when properly used, too often they are misunderstood or misused, according to NCI experts. They say the mistaken impression persists that a supplement such as wheat bran will suffice. Although wheat bran (the most widely available supplement) may improve bowel function, it may not offer the possible health benefits available in other forms of fiber.

CALCIUM AND SOYBEANS

Calcium is a mineral found in dark green, leafy vegetables and dairy products. Calcium helps prevent abnormal growth of colon cells in people who have polyps, small growths that increase the risk of colon cancer. Half of all Americans are deficient in their daily intake of calcium, a mineral now known to be highly effective in preventing colon cancer. Researchers at Memorial Sloan-Kettering and Cornell University Medical Center in New York found that dietary supplementation with calcium significantly reduced the proliferation of epithelial cells lining the colon within two to three months after supplementation. The overproduction of epithelial cells is often a forerunner of cancer and thus people at high risk for colon cancer can take calcium to help protect their colons against the development of malignancy.

Fiber, however, can remove essential minerals such as calcium, iron, and zinc from the body. Soybeans and many soybean products are rich in calcium and zinc, but how much the fiber in them may affect the minerals is still to be defined. Half a cup of soft tofu, for example, has no fiber and 130 milligrams of calcium. Half a cup of cooked soybeans has eighty-eight milligrams of calcium, 1 milligram of zinc, and 1.8 grams of fiber.

Summing it up, however, soybeans and other legumes are excellent in promoting healthy colons and bowel functions. They help protect against constipation, diverticular disease, hemorrhoids, and other bowel dysfunctions, and, if current research is confirmed, against colon cancer. They cannot do it alone and a well-balanced diet, low in fats and high in fruits and vegetables, will certainly help soy help you.

Chapter 4

How Soy Is Beneficial
in Diabetic Diets

Diabetes is a disease in which the body doesn't produce or properly use insulin. Insulin is needed to convert sugar and starch into the energy needed in daily life. Diabetics often suffer from high blood pressure and are more prone to suffering a heart attack or stroke than persons without the condition. The frequency of heart disease in diabetics is two to three times that of the general population.

Diabetes and complications from diabetes are the third major cause of death in the United States. Approximately 14 million people in the United States have diabetes. Approximately 25 percent of people with diabetes have type I, that is, insulin-dependent, whose bodies produce little or no insulin. Approximately 75 percent of the people with diabetes have type II, that is, non-insulin-dependent, whose bodies produce insulin but do not use it properly.

Type II, the more common form of the diabetes, usually occurs in overweight adults over age forty, and can often be treated with dietary changes and oral medications.

Glucose is a sugar that occurs naturally in blood, grapes, and corn. It is sweeter than sucrose, common table sugar. Until the 1980s, it was believed that sugar—a simple carbohydrate—raises blood glucose higher and faster than more complex carbohydrates, starches. Then data showed that chemically similar foods containing simple sugars and starches can in fact differ in their impact on blood sugar. It was discovered that even though a bowl of rice and a bowl of spaghetti may provide about the same nutrients, for some people the rice would raise the blood sugar higher and faster than the spaghetti. That is, the rice produces a higher "glycemic," or blood sugar, response. There is also a large difference in blood sugar elevations from ingestion of various foods between normal and diabetic people.

In 1981, Dr. David Jenkins at the University of Toronto published an article in the *American Journal of Clinical Nutrition* describing a glycemic index. It showed the different effects on blood sugar of various foods. Glucose—ordinary sugar—produces a blood sugar response rated at 100 percent in the index. By comparison, soybeans produce 10 to 20 percent. Brown rice has a 60 to 69 percent rating.

The index showed that legumes such as soybeans seem to be digested slowly and thus cause less of a rise in blood sugar. Unlike many legumes, however, soybeans do not contain significant quantities of starch. A study performed by G. S. Lo and his colleagues at Protein Technologies International in St. Louis and reported in *Advances in Experimental Medicine and Biology* showed that soy-fiber supplementation significantly reduced insulin response to oral glucose challenge by 20 percent in type II diabetics with high cholesterol and by 16.5 percent in those with high triglycerides (a type of blood fat).

Actually, the benefit of soy in the management of diabetes goes back to the early 1900s when Dr. John Kellogg, more famous for cornflakes than for soybeans, nevertheless wrote about the use of the bean in treating diabetes. Dr. Kellogg, who ran a sanitorium in Battle Creek, Michigan, accidentally developed a breakfast cereal while trying to concoct a more digestible bread for his patients. Cornflakes, of course, made Dr. Kellogg a multimillionaire and he promoted his ideas about vegetarianism with unrestrained vigor. Among the foods he recommended for diabetics were soybeans.

Several years before Dr. Kellogg's recommendation, two doctors, J. Friedenwald and J. Ruhrah, had prescribed soybeans as a food for diabetics in the *American Journal of Medical Science*.

Nearly four decades later, A. C. Tsai and colleagues performed a study of obese diabetic patients. The scientists reported in the *American Journal of Clinical Nutrition* the results of giving patients meals with or without ten grams of soy fiber. They found that those who developed diabetes as adults had their blood sugar levels return toward premeal level during the latter half of the meal test. The addition of soy fiber to the meal significantly reduced the rise of the eater's blood sugar and blood triglycerides (fats).

Unprocessed soy would have the best glycemic index rating of the soy products because processed foods are digested more quickly. Grinding, mashing, pureeing, and juicing all tend to promote higher blood sugar.

Soybeans also contain magnesium. Diabetes mellitus, which causes magnesium wasting, is marked by high blood fats and lesions of small blood vessels that resemble those seen in experiments or with magnesium deficiency. Magnesium deficiency may also occur in pregnancy, aging, or both physical and psychological stress.

Vegetarians in general have a much higher magnesium intake than meat eaters, which could be a factor in their lower incidence of heart and blood vessel disease.

James W. Anderson, M.D., professor of medicine and nutrition at the University of Kentucky, whose article on soy's capacity to lower cholesterol in the *New England*

Journal of Medicine on August 3, 1995, caused such a stir, at this writing has embarked on a soy and diabetes study.

Teresa Lancaster, clinical research assistant at the University of Kentucky's Metabolic Research Group, said the design of the study involves twelve patients who have had type II diabetes for five or more years, who are on insulin, and who have slight kidney involvement.

Jill Emmett, R.N., who is coordinating the study, said the participants are admitted to the hospital for a week at the start of each dietary change for careful monitoring. One group is on the regular diabetes diet with their protein from animal and dairy products. The other group is on the diabetes diet but with their protein derived from "soy meat" replacement and a powdered soy beverage. At the end of eight weeks, after thorough testing of their blood and urine, each group is again admitted to the hospital and goes on the opposite protocol: The ones with the animal protein in their diet will have soy protein instead and those on soy protein will have animal protein. Then Dr. Anderson and his group of Kentucky researchers will evaluate all their data and the effect of both diets on the diabetic patients.

Summing it up, type II diabetes can often be controlled completely by loss of weight, a diet high in fruits, grains, legumes, and vegetables, and exercising. Soybeans have already been shown to have a slow blood sugar response on the glycemic scale. They are also useful as a substitute for animal protein that reduces calorie intake. The question is now whether there is something in soybeans that may prove therapeutic in the treatment of diabetes.

Chapter 5

HOW SOY IS PROVING
BENEFICIAL TO WOMEN

Hormones, by definition, are chemical substances formed in one gland or part of the body and carried by the blood to another organ, which they stimulate to functional activity. The word *hormone* is actually from the Greek word *hormao,* meaning "I arouse to activity." The rise and fall of hormone levels in the female body greatly affect physical and emotional well-being.

In her whole life, a woman produces less than two teaspoonfuls of the female hormones estrogen and progesterone, yet the survival of the human race depends upon the release and perfect synchronization of microscopic amounts of these substances.

The word *estrogen* is derived from the Greek *oistros,* meaning "mad desire." No one claims that soybeans are an aphrodisiac, but like other legumes, they contain substantial amounts of plant estrogens called *isoflavones.* As pointed out in previous chapters, isoflavones are weaker than the human hormones but they aim for the same receptor sites on human cells and are believed to be able to block human estrogens in a sort of I-got-here-first-and-you-can't-play situation. Tamoxifen, isolated from a Pacific yew tree, and now widely used to treat breast cancer, does its work in this manner. It dampens human estrogen from stimulating breast cancer growth.

The problem with tamoxifen is that it may have side effects such as a drop in white blood count, weight gain, and bone pain. It may also cause uterine cancer after prolonged use.

How plant estrogens in soy and other foods work in the body may depend upon a woman's age, according to Johanna Dwyer and her colleagues at New England Medical Center and Tufts University. In an article in *The Journal of The American Dietetic Association,* July 1994, they theorize that in *pre*menopausal women who have high levels of circulating estrogen, the estrogen receptors (docking stations on the cell) are occupied and plant estrogens must compete for these sites. Because the plant estrogens have lower "docking" power than human-made estrogens, the net effect may be only weakly anti-estrogenic. In *post*menopausal women, however, the New England researchers say, self-produced estrogen concentration declines about 60 percent from premenopausal levels. Therefore, the chances of an estrogen "docking" site being unoccupied in an older woman's body are greater and plant estrogens, such as those in soybeans, can more easily find a place to anchor and thus increase the total amount of estrogens available to her. Consumption of foods containing phytoestrogens has been credited with contributing to the lower rate of menopausal symptoms among Japanese women compared with women in Western countries. Japanese women have much higher plant estrogen concentrations in their urine than Western women, as might be expected because of the high intake of whole soy foods.

At any age, soy in the diet may help prevent breast

cancer. One reason is that it lengthens the menstrual cycle, reducing a woman's body to some exposure to self-produced estrogens. Asian women, who have significantly fewer cycles than American women, also have the lowest breast cancer rates in the world.

THE SOY AND THE CYCLE

Researchers are now studying the effect of soybeans on the hormone levels of women with premenstrual syndrome and women who are postmenopausal. The latter become vulnerable to heart disease, cancer, and bone loss after their menses cease. Scientists want to determine if isoflavones, like human estrogens, can reduce the risks of heart disease, cancer, and fragile bones as well as alleviate the annoying symptoms of menopause.

Kenneth Setchell, Ph.D., professor of pediatrics at Children's Hospital and Medical Center in Cincinnati, demonstrated that regular soy foods contain enough plant estrogens to have a marked hormonal influence. He and his colleagues Aedin Cassidy and Sheila Bingham fed a group of young women sixty grams of textured soy protein daily and observed what happened to their menstrual cycles. After four weeks, the time between their cycles increased two to five days. Longer menstrual cycles mean a lower lifelong exposure to estrogen, which in turn is believed to lower cancer risk.

Dr. Setchell then tested whether oriental-style fermented soy foods such as miso (see page 95) and tempeh (see page 87) had a similar effect. He fed sixty grams of miso to volunteers. The miso had an even bigger effect. "It shifted the menstrual period an extra day," says Dr. Setchell, who now has a National Institutes of Health grant to study the physiological effects of the different soy estrogen compounds.

In several women, after the soy diet, three menstrual cycles elapsed before the cycle length returned to its original value.

The researchers reported their findings in the *American Journal of Clinical Nutrition* in 1994. They pointed out in their article:

> Recent and controversial trials of low doses of tamoxifen as a prophylactic agent are under way in women at high risk for breast cancer but with no evidence of the disease. This has been a controversial project because of the potentially serious side effects. The earlier demonstration that soy protein containing isoflavones have anticancer actions in animal models of breast cancer raises the question of whether dietary intervention with soy protein should be considered as an alternative to tamoxifen for breast cancer prevention.

In a study published in 1995 in the *Journal of Clinical Endocrinology and Metabolism* in which Dr. Setchell also participated along with Donna Day Baird of the Epidemiology Branch of the National Institute of Environmental Health Sciences, Claude Hughes of the Bowman Gray School of Medicine in Winston-Salem, North Carolina, and others, postmenopausal women were given a soy-supplemented diet to test their estrogen responses. Ninety-seven women were randomized to either a group that was provided with soy foods for four weeks or to a control group that was instructed to eat as usual. Those who ate soy ingested 165 milligrams per day of isoflavones.

Changes in urinary isoflavone concentration (soybean estrogen) served as a measure of compliance and phytoestrogen dose. Changes in sex hormones in the blood and vaginal cells were measured to assess estrogen response. The percentage of vaginal superficial cells—indicative of estrogen response—increased for 19 percent for those eating the diet compared with 8 percent of controls. Little change occurred in the women's own self-produced estrogen or in their body weight during the diet.

The researchers said that based on published estimates of phytoestrogen potency, a four-week soy-supplemented diet was expected to have estrogenic effects on the liver and pituitary in postmenopausal women, but such effects were not seen. At most, there was a small estrogen effect on vaginal cells.

The investigators said in summary that this was the first intervention study of postmenopausal women to measure urinary levels of phytoestrogens. The response was weaker than expected, but the scientists concluded that more sensitive tests and a longer period of time may be necessary to evaluate the effects of soybean estrogens in postmenopausal women.

OTHER HORMONAL BENEFITS

Genistein, as mentioned in Chapter 2, is perhaps the most important soybean estrogen. The plant hormones, it is believed, may ease diseases like rheumatoid arthritis, psoriasis, and diabetic retinopathy (eye damage).

Genistein at the lowest dose had a similar effect as Premarin in maintaining trabecular bone tissue, but at the higher doses it had essentially no retentive effect on bone tissue, according to a study by Dr. J. J. Anderson and his colleagues in the Department of Nutrition and Dental Research at the University of North Carolina in Chapel Hill.

Daidzein, another plant estrogen found in soybeans, is now also under intensive study. Like genistein, it is turned by intestinal bacteria into a substance that competes with human estrogen. Along with genistein, daidzein is being intensively studied for its potential cancer-preventive capacity.

Cooking, baking, or frying do not seem to affect phytoestrogens. The following table shows amounts of these two plant phytoestrogens in some soy products.

PHYTOESTROGENS: WHERE TO FIND THEM

PRODUCT	DAIDZEIN MG/KG	GENISTEIN MG/KG
Soybeans (dried)	1001.3	1022.7
Soybeans (fresh)	252.0	257.0
Soy flour	654.7	1122.6
Tofu	113.4	166.4
Miso	79.0	177.0
Black soybeans (boiled)	273.0	277.1
Bean paste	272.0	245.0
Fermented bean curd	143.0	224.0
Tempeh	273.0	245.0
Green split peas (dry)	72.6	not detectable

Reprinted with permission from: A. A. Franke, L. J. Custer, C. M. Cerna, and K. K. Narala, "Quantitation of Phytoestrogens in Legumes by HPLC," *Journal of Agricultural Food Chemistry.* 42: 1905–13, 1994.

MAGNESIUM, PMS, AND PREGNANCY

It is not just the isoflavones in soy that may have a beneficial effect on the menstrual cycle, magnesium may also have some effect. Magnesium, which is high in soybeans, has been reported beneficial to women with premenstrual syndrome, according to a 1994 study by D. L. Rosenstein and his colleagues at the National Institute of Mental Health in Bethesda, Maryland, and reported in *Biological Psychiatry*. The researchers found that twenty-six women with confirmed PMS had decreased red blood cell magnesium. Low magnesium levels have also been reported in chronic fatigue syndrome (CFS) by I. M. Cox and his colleagues at the University of South Hampton Medical School in Britain in the British medical journal *Lancet*. CFS is a common and frequently debilitating illness, the cause or causes of which are still unknown. The researchers found that patients with CFS have low red blood cell magnesium. Fifteen patients with CFS were treated with magnesium and twelve improved significantly. In a not uncommon situation, the Irish do not agree with the British. Dr. G. Hinds and his colleagues at Queen's University's Department of Medicine in Northern Ireland measured the red blood cell magnesium concentration in eighty-nine patients with CFS. In their report in the *Annals of Clinical Biochemistry*, they maintained they found no significant difference in the magnesium blood levels between patients with and without CFS.

Less controversial than magnesium and CFS is the importance of the mineral in pregnancy. Dr. R. Zarcone and his colleagues at the Institute of Gynecology and Obstetrics, Second University of Naples, Italy, reported in *Panminerva Medicine* in 1994 a study of women at high risk of giving birth prematurely. Half were given magnesium supplementation and half were not. Many more of the control group women were admitted to the hospital for premature labor than were those given magnesium supplementation.

Magnesium can be toxic in high doses so supplementation in pregnancy should be done only with professional advice.

CONTRACEPTIVE OR FERTILITY INDUCER?

The idea that soybeans may interfere with fertility came into being with two animal studies. The first dramatic example occurred in Southwest Australia when the sheep-breeding industry was decimated because the sheep were infertile. It was discovered that the red clover on which the animals grazed contained levels of isoflavones high enough to make the animals sterile. The second incident occurred at the Cincinnati Zoo where cheetahs were not reproducing and developed liver problems. Researchers found that the standard cat chow given big cats was about half soybean product, thus dosing the felines with a rather high level of plant estrogens. When the soybeans were replaced with meat from chickens, the cheetahs displayed signs of increased fertility and other hormone-related activity.

Mark Messina, Ph.D., a leading authority on soybeans and health, decries the idea that the fertility of women may be adversely affected by eating soy foods. He points out that in Japan and China women eat a high level of soy foods and have no trouble with their fertility.

Dr. Setchell agrees: "The critical issue that people fail to realize is that although soy lengthens the cycle, it doesn't actually prevent ovulation. There is no effect on progesterone and there is still a normal menstrual cycle."

Both Drs. Messina and Setchell say that any individual can have a stronger reaction to a substance than the population at large, but as long as a woman maintains regular periods, there is no reason to stop eating soy for fear that it will interfere with conception.

SO "B" IT

Soybeans also contain pantothenic acid, a B vitamin that may be beneficial against many conditions of concern to women, such as digestive disorders, mood swings, and headaches. Pantothenic acid stimulates adrenal glands, aids cellular metabolism, helps metabolize cholesterol and fatty acids, and helps maintain a healthy digestive tract. It may help prevent birth defects, mental fatigue, sleep disturbances, headaches, muscle spasms, and breathing problems.

The recommended daily intake is ten milligrams. Overdoing the intake of pantothenic acid, however, may cause diarrhea and water retention. Food processing, sleeping pills, alcohol, tobacco, caffeine, and estrogen can destroy pantothenic acid in soybeans or other foods containing this B vitamin.

THE BONES NEED IT

Osteoporosis is a condition characterized by low bone mass and an increased susceptibility to bone fractures. The adult body contains about three pounds of calcium, 99 percent of which provides hardness for bones and teeth. Approximately 1 percent of calcium is distributed in body fluids, where it is essential for normal cell activity. If the body does not get enough calcium from food, it steals the mineral from bones. Abnormal loss of calcium from bones weakens them, making them porous or brittle and susceptible to fractures. Calcium deficiencies can result in osteopenia (less bone than normal), a condition preceding osteoporosis (a severe decrease in bone mass with diagnosable fractures) that affects 25 percent of women after menopause. The percentage of calcium absorption declines progressively with age. There is some evidence that an intake of about 1000 milligrams of calcium may protect against hypertension or high blood pressure.

A panel of experts convened by the National Institutes of Health recommended in June 1994 that most Americans increase their daily intake of calcium to prevent osteoporosis. The recommended dietary allowance for calcium is 1000 milligrams for adults.

Although soybeans are high in calcium, there is a question about how much can be absorbed. Soybeans contain phytic acid, which may interfere with the absorption of calcium. However, research suggests that replacing some animal protein with soy protein slows calcium loss by a third. Ounce for ounce, for example, tofu made with calcium has as much or more calcium than a glass of milk. One-half cup of natto (see page 97) has 191 milligrams of calcium, 24 percent of the RDA, and one cup of EdenSoy brand soy milk has 20 percent of the RDA.

MAGNESIUM AND BONES

Soybeans, as pointed out several times in this book, contain magnesium. Magnesium regulates active calcium transport through the body. As a result, there has been a growing interest in the role of magnesium in bone metabolism. Drs. J. E. Sojka and C. M. Weaver of Purdue University conducted a study of a group of menopausal women. The subjects were given magnesium hydroxide to assess the effects of the mineral on bone density. At the end of the two-year study, according to the researchers report in *Nutrition Review* in 1995, magnesium therapy appeared to have prevented fractures and resulted in a significant increase in bone density.

BORON AND BONES

Since the early 1980s, evidence has been accumulating that the trace element boron is necessary for animal health. It was long thought necessary for plant life. In 1981, researchers reported that boron deprivation depressed growth and elevated blood alkaline phosphate activity in chicks. In a 1986 study done by Forrest Nielsen, Ph.D., director of the U.S. Department of Agriculture's Agricultural Research Center in Grand Forks, North Dakota, of postmenopausal women between the ages of forty-eight and eighty-two years, the women were given three milligrams of boron per day. The boron markedly affected the metabolism of seven women consuming a low-magnesium diet and five women consuming a diet adequate in magnesium. Boron supplementation markedly reduced the urinary excretion of calcium and magnesium. The boron supplementation also raised the level of estradiol-17 beta, a female hormone, and testosterone, a male hormone. The changes in the hormone concentration were particularly noteworthy because estradiol-17 beta is the most biologically active form of human estrogen, and estrogen administration is the only known effective means to slow the loss of calcium from bone that occurs after menopause. Testosterone is a precursor of estradiol-17 beta. During this study, reported in the January/February 1988 issue of *Nutrition Today,* two women were on estrogen therapy; their serum estradiol-17 beta levels were the same as the women fed supplemental boron without estrogen therapy. Like the animal studies, the findings indicate that boron deprivation leads to suboptimal mineral metabolism. In fact, boron may be an important nutritional factor determining the incidence of osteoporosis. Foods of plant origin, including soybeans, are rich sources of boron. Meat or fish are apparently poor sources of boron.

IT COULD BE THE PHYTATES

In plants, phytate is the storage form of the mineral phosphorus, which is necessary for every tissue in the body, but especially bone. In fact, 85 percent of our body's phosphorus—about twenty ounces—is found in bone. It accounts for 6 percent of bone material. Phytates are known to bind calcium and iron in the intestines and carry them out of the body before they can be absorbed.

Since soybeans are high in phytate, they were thought to be destructive to bone strength. Scientists have long believed that since phosphorus and calcium are partners, they should be equal—one to one. They theorized that a higher phosphorus ratio in the body caused demineralization of the bone, but now they are not so sure. In fact, many believe that phosphorus supplements may help calcium be retained. Some research has shown that phosphorus may reduce both the pain of arthritis and the effects of stress. Phytates are high in soybeans and other foods that have a lot of fiber, and may help, not hinder, bone strength.

The phytoestrogens genistein and daidzein are also believed to help protect women against bone loss if their intake is sufficient and prolonged.

Whether or not soybeans can significantly add to the prevention of osteoporosis in postmenopausal women isn't definitive yet, but the boron, calcium, and magnesium they contain as well as the phytoestrogens and phytates certainly seem to indicate they can. The scientific proof is yet to come.

Chapter 6

SOY AND MEN

Like other wives, Hillary Clinton worries about her man's health, especially when her husband, the president, loves to eat hamburgers and French fries. The first lady has arranged to have hamburgers in the White House and on *Air Force One,* but instead of fat-ladened beefy ones, the patties are made of soy-based protein. A soy-based hamburger contains:

- 84 to 110 calories
- 0 to 2 grams of fat
- 0 cholesterol
- 4 to 5 grams of fiber

A fast-food hamburger, on the other hand, which the president likes to sneak when he can, contains:

- 272 calories
- 11 grams of fat
- 37 milligrams of cholesterol
- 0 fiber

There is no report about whether Hillary has been able to scuttle the high-fat French fries, though, but males, including a president, do have a big stake in soy research. Men really are the weaker sex when it comes to taking care of their health. If you doubt it, consider these statistics:

- Men suffer from 100,000 more cancers per year than women.
- Men develop coronary artery disease ten to fifteen years earlier than women.
- Men are less likely than women to change their eating habits to help their health and average only three servings of fruits and vegetables a day while women have four (health experts recommend five or more servings).
- Men usually have no prescribed routine health care and unless there is a request for a sports, army, insurance, or annual company physical, there is usually no structure in which men can be followed medically.
- Men are less likely to heed their doctor's advice and to return for a checkup after they have been ill.
- Women buy most of the books and magazines about health.

It is no wonder then that more males than females die at every decade of life. By age sixty-five, women outnumber men three to two and at eighty-five, they outnumber men five to two.

This is true in America but how about Japan where the men's diets are high in soy foods? Japanese men are among the longest lived males in the world. The average life expectancy for them is 82.5 years, according to UN statistics, while for the American male, it is about seventy-two years. Epidemiological studies show that in the Orient the consumption of soy foods is twenty to fifty times greater than in the United States.

No one can say it is just because of the soy in the Japanese diet. One outstanding example of the difference between American and Japanese men's health, however, is the rate of their prostate problems and the variation has been associated with soy intake.

The prostate is a walnut-sized gland in the male pelvis that produces fluid that helps to nourish and transport sperm. Most American men, if they live long enough, will find they have problems urinating because of an enlarged prostate. This condition, known as benign prostate hyperplasia (BPH), is characterized by hesitant and slow urination flow and frequent urination at night, interfering with sleep. The American Cancer Society, in addition, estimates that 18.54 percent of American men will also develop prostate cancer in their lives. In one year, it will be diagnosed in 317,000 men and claim the lives of 41,400. Death rates from prostate cancer, adjusted for age, have been rising steadily since 1930, and are especially high among American blacks, according to National Cancer Institute statistics.

The soy in the Japanese diet apparently helps to protect the prostate gland. A low mortality from prostatic cancer is found in Japanese men consuming a low-fat diet with a high content of soy products, according to H. Adlercreutz and his colleagues at the University of Helsinki in Finland. They checked four plant estrogens in the blood of fourteen Japanese and fourteen Finnish men. They found the levels were 7 to 110 times higher in the Japanese than in the Finns. Genistein, a reportedly beneficial soybean estrogen, occurred in the highest concentration. The Finnish researchers hypothesized that these high phytoestrogen levels may inhibit the growth of prostatic cancer in Japanese men, which they said may explain the low mortality from prostatic cancer in that country.

Similar hope for the preventive powers of genistein,

the soy phytoestrogen, against prostate cancer evolves in the laboratory of Dr. Lothar Schweigerer and his colleagues at Heidelberg University. They discovered, as pointed out earlier, that genistein blocks an event called angiogenesis, the growth of new blood vessels that nourish malignant tumors. Once a tumor grows beyond a millimeter, it must foster the growth of new blood vessels around it. When it is fully vascularized, the malignancy then receives the oxygen and nourishment it needs to grow and to eventually send fatal metastatic colonies elsewhere. By inhibiting blood vessel growth, genistein may keep new tumors from growing beyond harmless dimensions. This could also explain why, when Japanese men leave their country for several years to work in the United States or Europe, their rate of invasive prostate cancer rises sharply. Dr. Schweigerer postulates that tiny prostate tumors that had been kept in check by daily intake of, say, miso soup, would finally be free to grow once the Japanese men ate a more Western diet.

William Fair, M.D., chief of urology, and Warren Heston, M.D., of Memorial Sloan-Kettering Cancer Center in New York City, in collaboration with the American Health Foundation, are conducting a dietary study in men who have undergone radical surgery for prostate cancer. Half the men are consuming a normal diet of 40 percent of calories from fat. The others are on a diet containing only 15 percent of calories from fat. In addition, each day the treatment group will consume two protein shakes containing a 50-milligram supplement of vitamin E and four-tenths of a milligram of selenium.

Dr. Fair told Jane Brody of the *New York Times,* October 18, 1995, that in animal studies, "soy protein has looked almost as good as a low-fat diet in slowing the progression of prostate cancer." Both vitamin E and selenium are antioxidants that a few studies have suggested may counter prostate trouble.

"We don't expect that a prostate tumor will be eliminated by this diet but it might be able to delay its progression by as much as thirty years," Dr. Fair told the *Times*. He emphasized that the diet is not a substitute for standard therapy. "Rather it is an addition to it that may be especially appropriate for men with a strong family history of prostate cancer and men with an elevated PSA level [a diagnostic test for prostate cancer] as well as men who have already been treated for prostate cancer."

Dr. Fair said that "while more research is needed to convince the scientific community of the diet's benefits, there is nothing wrong with going on it, since the downside is essentially zero."

Genistein in soybeans is now also being tested against Kaposi's sarcoma, a cancer frequently linked to AIDS, a terrible disease currently affecting predominantly males.

Ironically, pharmaceutical statisticians are predicting that the largest increase in cancers—including colon, breast, and prostate—will be in Japan in the future because the Japanese diet is becoming more westernized, including increasing amounts of animal fats and calories. The incidence and mortality rates for cancers is already showing an upswing in Japan.

One of the cancers increasing among Japanese men is colon cancer, the third most common cancer plaguing men in the United States. According to the American Cancer Society, more than 67,600 American men this year will be diagnosed with bowel malignancies and 27,400 will die of them.

An American Cancer Society study analyzed by Michael Thun, M.D., director of analytical epidemiology for the American Cancer Society, reported on a large study of colon cancer and diet in 1992. The prospective study uses data from the Society's Cancer Prevention Study II

(CPS II) to assess the relation of diet and other factors to risk of fatal colon cancer. CPS II is an ongoing mortality study started in 1982 that analyzed the diet, behavior, and lifestyles of 1,185,124 American men and women through the use of questionnaires. It is one of the largest research studies ever carried out in the United States.

Dr. Thun and his colleagues' findings revealed that men who consumed the least vegetables and grains and no aspirin had a 2.5 times higher risk of colon cancer compared to those who consumed the most vegetables and used low-dose aspirin sixteen or more times a month.

The results support recommendations by the American Cancer Society and the U.S. Department of Health and Human Services encouraging consumption of a variety of vegetables, fruits, and high-fiber grains.

As you have read in Chapter 2, Geoffrey Howe, Jr., M.D., of the University of Toronto found that in twelve of thirteen studies, eating lots of fiber in foods can indeed slash the risk of colon cancer about in half. Dr. Howe and colleagues figure that if everyone ate about 70 percent more fiber than usual, the rates of colon and rectal cancers would drop 31 percent, preventing an annual 50,000 new cases in both men and women of all ages.

This would mean adding at least thirteen grams of food fiber daily for most people, about the amount in a serving of two soy-based burgers—the kind Hillary has at the White House. Soy, as you have read in Chapter 3, also contains other cancer-fighting substances.

SOY AND SEX

In some cases, it is possible that the phytoestrogens in soy-beans may help men with a fertility problem. Antiestrogens such as tamoxifen, which block the body's own self-produced estrogen from activity, affect the blood levels of LH (luteinizing hormone) needed for normal sperm production. Tamoxifen (Nolvadex®), originally derived from the bark of a Pacific yew tree, is widely used to treat breast cancer and was reported in 1995 to be successful in preventing some breast cancers. Genistein, the phytoestrogen in soy, is believed to have an antiestrogen effect similar to tamoxifen and may be of use in treating male sterility since it has less side effects than tamoxifen. Japanese men eat between forty and seventy milligrams of genistein per day. American men eat less than one milligram per day.

The zinc in soybeans may also be beneficial to men. Soybeans are a good source of zinc, a mineral used by the body in the formation of many hormones. It also functions as an antioxidant. Zinc deficiency has been found to affect reproduction in animals. Although not proven, zinc has also been reputed to increase male potency and sex drive.

PROTEIN POWER

Many men—especially young athletes—believe that additional protein will power their muscles. The proteins we eat are used by our bodies to build new tissue and repair damaged cells, it is true, but an overdose of protein can adversely affect the kidneys.

Proteins are among the most complicated of molecules. They are employed by our bodies to make hormones, enzymes, and neurotransmitters, the brain's chemical messengers. Proteins keep the acid/alkaline content in our blood in balance, and collect and dispose of waste products. Those proteins that are not immediately used are stored in fat.

The Committee on Dietary Guidelines Implementation of the Food and Nutrition Board at the National Institute of Medicine says that according to a national survey, men from ages nineteen to fifty consume an average of ninety-eight grams of protein per day. Approximately two-thirds of the protein comes from animal products and one-third from plants. The NIM committee recommends that protein intake *not* be increased (see the chart below) but that the intake of meat and dairy products be limited to six ounces or less per day. The rest of the protein needed can be made up by the ingestion of soy and other vegetable products.

RDAs FOR PROTEIN AND MAXIMUM RECOMMENDED INTAKES FOR MEN

CATEGORY	AGE	RDA G/KG	MEDIAN WEIGHT IN LBS	RDA G/DAY	MAXIMUM G/DAY
Males	11–14	1.0	99	45	90
	15–18	0.9	145	59	118
	19–24	0.8	158	58	116
	25+	0.8	173	63	126

A change in men's diet—increasing the intake of soy, fruits, and vegetables while reducing meat and dairy products—can, as you have read in this book, reduce their incidence of cancer, heart and blood vessel disease, and prostate problems. It is believed by many eminent researchers that such a change will increase American men's years of life and make those years more lively.

Chapter 7

SOY PRODUCTS AND
THEIR NUTRITIONAL VALUE

You have many choices of soy foods today in your super-market and health food store. There are those concocted in traditional ways and typically divided into two categories: *nonfermented* and *fermented*.

During the past decade, 2000 new soy products have also made their way into the food stores. They not only make interesting additions to our diet, as you have read in this book, but they also have health benefits known and yet to be discovered. Soybeans can be used green or dry. The nutrition value of one half cup of hulled green soybeans has the same protein content as an eight-ounce glass of milk. The iron content is the same as two eggs, while providing about one-half the daily vitamin C requirement for adults.

Cooked soybeans contain 23 percent of the recommended daily allowance of folacin, 22 percent of the RDA for calcium, 49 percent for iron, and 53 percent for phosphorus.

Dried soybeans are also a good value. One half-cup serving of cooked dried soybeans contains the protein of a two-ounce serving of meat, the iron equivalent of three eggs, and the calcium equivalent of a half cup of milk.

The following is a short primer on the major types of soy products available and their nutritional values.

SOYBEANS

Fresh soybeans can be hard to find in some areas. Sunrich, a midwestern distributor, has rechristened mature fresh soybeans "sweet beans" and has been taste-marketing them in the Minneapolis-St. Paul area, reportedly with good results. Green soybeans can be cooked like lima beans or peas. Fresh soybeans have all the health benefits of other soy products; in addition they're high in fiber.

If you have a problem with "gas" or flatulence when you eat beans, it is because your body cannot break down the complex sugars raffinose and stachyose. These sugars sit in the gut and are fermented by intestinal bacteria that then produce gas, which can distend our intestines and makes us uncomfortable. You can lessen this effect by covering the beans with water, boiling the water for three minutes, and then soaking the beans for from four to six hours. Throw the water away. (You may somewhat reduce the nutrients and protein in the beans.) Add new water and cook the beans. Drain them before serving. Preprocessed dried soybeans take less time to cook but they are lower in B vitamins. You may also wish to obtain Beano in your health food store or by calling Beano at 1-800-257-8650 (in Canada, call 1-800-668-8968). This product contains an enzyme that helps avoid a gas problem caused by beans.

Canning destroys some of the B vitamins in soybeans. Since the B vitamins are water soluble, you could save them by using the liquid in the can. But the liquid may also contain the indigestible sugars that cause intestinal gas when you eat beans.

You should store soybeans in airtight moistureproof containers in a cool dark cabinet where they are protected from light, heat, and insects.

EDAMAME

These are young soybeans, which are salted and cooked until tender. A Japanese specialty, they are sold in pods, shelled, canned, or frozen.

NUTRIENTS IN ½ CUP GREEN SOYBEANS WITHOUT PODS*

Calories	60
Total fat	2 g
Saturated fat	1 g
Unsaturated fat	1 g
Carbohydrate	3 g
Fiber	8 g
Thiamine	0.5 mg
Calcium	40 mg
Vitamin C	10 mg
Sugar	3 g
Protein	6 g

*See Sources, page 103.

NUTRIENTS IN ½ CUP COOKED SOYBEANS*

Calories	149
Protein	14.3 g
Total fat	7.7 g
Saturated fat	1.1 g
Unsaturated fat	6.6 g

Carbohydrate	8.5 g
Fiber	1.8 g
Calcium	88 mglron
Iron	4.4 mg
Zinc	1.0 mg
Thiamine	0.1 mg
Riboflavin	0.3 mg
Vitamin C	.21 mg
Niacin	0.3 mg
Vitamin B_6	0.2 mg
Folacin	46.2 mg

*See Sources, page 103.

SOYBEAN SPROUTS

Soybean sprouts are nutritious and delicious and a bargain in folate, magnesium, and vitamin C. Unlike a number of soybean products, they are also low in sodium.

NUTRIENTS IN ½ CUP RAW SOYBEAN SPROUTS*

Calories	45
Total fat	2.5 g
Saturated fat	0.3 g
Monounsaturated fat	0.3 g
Polyunsaturated fat	1.3 g
Calories from fat	47%
Cholesterol	0
Sodium	5 mg
Protein	4.6 g
Carbohydrate	3.9 g
Fiber	N/A
Folate	60.1 mcg

Vitamin C	5.4 mg
Thiamine	0.1 mg
Iron	0.7 mg
Magnesium	25.2 mg

*See Sources, page 103.

TOFU
(ALSO KNOWN AS BEAN CURD AND DOU FU-TOFU)

The Chinese called tofu "meat without bones" or "meat of the fields" because it is rich in protein and minerals. A Chinese ruler, Lui An, is credited with creating tofu in 200 B.C. Buddhist monks took soybeans from China to Japan between the sixth and eighth centuries. When the monks opened vegetarian restaurants in their temples in the twelfth century, Japanese laymen ate their first tofu. It first made inroads into the American market in the 1980s. Tofutti, an ice cream substitute made from tofu, became a hit within two years.

Tofu contains high levels of the phytoestrogen daidzein. Johanna Dwyer, director of the nutrition center at the New England Medical Center in Boston, and her colleagues discovered that different brands of tofu contain anywhere from seventy-three to ninety-seven micrograms of daidzein in each gram. As tofu intake increases in the American diet, daidzein may help prevent breast cancer (see Chapter 3).

In much the same way that cheese is made from animal milk, tofu is made from soy milk curds. Tofu is the result of adding a coagulant to soy milk, which separates it into curds and whey. The curds are compressed into soft, spongy blocks. Tofu is sold in many forms:

Firm. Pressed so there is less moisture and a relatively high concentration of nutrients. Must be refrigerated.

Regular. Softer and more delicate in texture. Must be refrigerated.

Soft. Slightly sweeter with a higher water content. Flavored for desserts. Must be refrigerated.

Silken. Also sweeter with a custardlike texture. Usually packaged in shelf-stable aseptic boxes.

Smoked. Usually precooked in a soy sauce–based seasoning, then smoked to achieve a browned surface, pleasant flavor, and firm, cheeselike texture. May have to be kept under refrigeration.

Dried. A freeze-dried product that is stored at room temperature and reconstituted with boiling water. Has a chewy texture and is useful for traveling and camping.

Tofu Pouches *or Age* (pronounced *AH-gay*). Deep-fried cubes of tofu that are hollow inside. Must be kept in the refrigerator or freezer.

Frozen. Freezing may change the texture from soft to chewy, but that may be acceptable if it means you always have some tofu on hand.

Tofu commonly comes in 10.25-ounce bricks in the supermarket produce aisle, although sometimes larger packages are available; the cost is between $1 to $1.50. Firm and soft tofu are for cooking; silken tofu, which has a custardlike texture, works best for blending. Natural food stores offer more textures and lower-fat options in the same price range.

You must be careful in selecting tofu if you buy it floating in water. There may be high levels of certain *E. coli,* a bacterium that can make you sick. You are better off buying it in sealed packages and then cooking it at a high temperature until it reaches 160°F. internally. Vacuum-packed fresh tofu can be kept for three to five weeks under refrigeration. Some companies are pasteurizing the tofu as well to extend this time and to allow for nationwide distribution. Be sure to check the expiration date on the wrapper. Tofu also comes canned in water and salt. The silken variety may be aseptically packaged and subjected to ultrahigh temperature sterilization, just like similarly packed milk and juice. The product then has a room temperature shelf life of three to six months.

Tofu is ordinarily highly perishable, so keep it under refrigeration. When bought in bulk or removed from its sealed package, it is best stored in a covered container submerged in water, which should be changed daily. Use as soon as possible or within one to three weeks of manufacture.

Fresh tofu is odorless and has a smooth but not slick surface. If either of these characteristics change (that is, if it begins to smell or develop a slippery texture), it is probably spoiling. Remember the tried-and-true saying about preventing foodborne illness: "When in doubt, throw it out!"

Tofu is high in protein and calcium providing as much, ounce for ounce, as skim milk. A little of the fat in tofu is saturated, the kind linked to cholesterol buildup, but most of it is unsaturated. *Firm* and *extrafirm* versions of tofu have more water removed. To get the forty-seven grams of protein through food, as the cholesterol studies indicate is therapeutic, you would have to eat three pounds of tofu—which contains sixteen grams of protein a pound—a day. Of course, it can be used many ways. It can be blended into drinks and dips, for instance. Swirled with frozen peaches, honey, and vanilla, *silken* tofu makes a light and frothy beverage. Folded into guacamole, tofu produces a cloudlike dip with less fat. (But contrary to popular perception, tofu is not very low in fat, which accounts for about half its calories; there are now "lower" fat tofus on the market.)

NUTRIENTS IN ½ CUP TOFU*

	FIRM TOFU	SOFT TOFU	SILKEN TOFU
Calories	120	86	72
Protein	13 g	9 g	9.6 g
Carbohydrate	3 g	2 g	3.2 g
Total fat	6 g	5 g	2.4 g
Saturated fat	1 g	1 g	0
Cholesterol	0	0	0
Sodium	9 mg	8 mg	76 mg
Fiber	1 g	0	0
Calcium	120 mg	130 mg	40 mg
Iron	8 mg	7 mg	1 mg
% of calories from protein	43	39	53
% of calories from carbohydrate	10	9	17
% of calories from fat	45	52	30

*See Sources, page 103.

TEMPEH

Tempeh—pronounced *TEM-pay*—is one of the most accessible, if exotic-sounding, soy products. Unlike tofu, it has a pleasant toothy texture. It is made from whole cooked soybeans infused with a "starter" and allowed to ferment in a mold, *Rhizopus,* from the hibiscus plant. Compressed into dense blocks, it has a chewy texture that is comparable to pecans or walnuts. Tempeh has a translucent, mushroomlike flavor. A three-ounce serving has about 150 calories (fifty from fat), sixteen grams of protein, and 6 grams of fiber. It is often used in grilling and stir-frying. Tempeh is low in soy protein and can be high in sodium. It may look unappealing, with flecks of gray or black spots, but that means it is just naturally fermented. The fermentation of the soybean during tempeh manufacture improves the protein and B vitamin content. This includes B_{12}, which usually only occurs in animals. Moreover, the iron and zinc in the tempeh are easily assimilated in the body. The fermentation also takes away the gas-producing bacteria so it is essentially nonflatulent. In fact, during World War II in a Japanese prison camp in the Philippines, the prisoners found boiled soybeans hard to digest. Several Dutch prisoners from Indonesia, who were familiar with tempeh, suggested fermentation. After obtaining a microbial culture, the men soaked the beans and fermented them outdoors in the hot climate. The resulting product was "successfully used in treating protein and vitamin deficiencies," according to a British medical report. Tempeh also contains a significant level of phytoestrogens. (See page 67.)

Tempeh can go a lot of places meat goes—for instance, between two slices of bread with tomato, lettuce, and

NUTRIENTS IN ½ CUP TEMPEH*

Calories	204
Protein	17 g
Total fat	8 g
Saturated fat	0.9 g
Monounsaturated fat	1.4 g
Polyunsaturated fat	3.6 g
Cholesterol	0
Sodium	5 mg
Carbohydrate	15 g
Calcium	80 mg
Iron	2 mg
Folate	42 mcg
Potassium	304.5 mg
Magnesium	58.1 mg
Zinc	1.5 mg

*See Sources, page 103.

mayonnaise—but it's not a meat substitute per se. Because tempeh is made from whole soybeans, it is high in fiber.

Believed to have originated in Indonesia more than 2000 years ago, tempeh is sold frozen, often in patties, at natural food stores for $1.50 to $2 for six ounces and thaws in about two minutes in the microwave. Marinate it before grilling, sautéing, or frying. In its dry state, it will keep for as long as a week.

SOY MILK

A combination of ground soybeans and water often used like dairy milk for drinking and cooking, soy milk is used as a base for tofu, soy yogurt, and soy-based cheeses. It is sold in health food stores and is available in whole and low-fat versions as well as flavored and plain varieties. One cup has about 4 percent protein.

Slightly nutty-tasting, the cappuccino-colored beverage has a texture similar to low-fat cows' milk. It is extracted from soybeans.

Soy milk is sold in various forms and flavors—low-

NUTRIENTS IN 1 CUP PLAIN SOY MILK*

	REGULAR SOY MILK	REDUCED-FAT SOY MILK
Calories	140	100
Protein	10 g	4 g
Fat	4 g	2 g
Carbohydrate	14 g	16 g
Sodium	120 mg	100 mg
Iron	1.8 mg	0.6 mg
Riboflavin	0.1 mg	0.11 mg
Calcium	80 mg	80 mg

*See Sources, page 103.

fat, vitamin-fortified, plain, vanilla, and carob—at natural food stores in aseptic, shelf-stable cartons that do not need refrigeration. A package of three single-serving cartons costs about $2.25.

Soy milk is rich in iron, phosphorus, thiamine, copper, potassium, and magnesium and is a good source of vegetable-quality protein. It is low in sugar, saturated fat, and sodium plus it can be ingested by people who have a problem with lactose, milk sugar. The following is the nutrition rundown on an eight-fluid-ounce serving of Eden-Soy Extra Original Soy Milk.

EDENSOY EXTRA ORIGINAL SOY MILK

Calories	130
from fat	35
Total fat	4 g
Saturated fat	0.5 g
Cholesterol	0
Sodium	105 mg
Potassium	440 mg
Total carbohydrate	13 g
Dietary fiber	0
Sugar	7 g
Protein	10 g
Vitamin A	30% of daily value
Calcium	20% of daily value
Vitamin E	10% of daily value
Thiamine (B_1)	10% of daily value
Niacin (B_3)	4% of daily value
Pantothenic acid (B_5)	6% of daily value
Pyridoxine hydrochloride (B_6)	8% of daily value
Folate (B_9)	10% of daily value
Vitamin B_{12}	50% of daily value
Phosphorus	15% of daily value

Magnesium	15% of daily value
Zinc	6% of daily value
Biotin (vitamin H)	4% of daily value

YUBA

Yuba, popular in Japan and China, is the "skin" that forms on hot soybean milk during processing. It is sold only in gourmet shops in Japan, but it is widely available in China. The Chinese often make yuba into imitation meat. Fresh yuba is pressed into molds made in the shape of various animals or parts of animals such as ducks' heads or fish and heated. When the animal-shaped product is unmolded, it is flavored and served cold, fried, or simmered in a broth. The meatless product is sold under traditional names such as Buddha's Duck and Molded Pig's Head. Yuba is 52.4 percent protein; it can be used in soups and stews.

SOY CHEESE

A relatively new category of cheese products on the market, soy cheese is low in calories and overall fat content. It is both lactose- and cholesterol-free and the sodium content is about average for dairy cheeses. Soy cheese is held together with vegetable gums and will contain either the milk derivative calcium caseinate, which is not dairy-free, or isolated soy protein (ISP), which is dairy-free.

OKARA

This is the pulp that remains when soy milk is strained. The word *okara* means "honorable hull." It has less protein than the whole bean but is still a good source of protein and fiber, and recent studies have shown it helps to lower cholesterol significantly. It has a coconut-like texture and is used in granola and cookies. It is also used in commercial vegetarian burgers. It is very perishable so you should keep it in the refrigerator and use it within a few days.

SOY YOGURT

Soy yogurt is cultured from soy milk. Active bacteria cultures are used but the yogurt is lactose- and cholesterol-free. It can be used in place of dairy yogurts in drinks, shakes, snacks, and desserts.

SOY SAUCE

The most widely recognized of soy foods is the sauce made from soybeans, wheat flour, and fermenting agents, such as yeast (for about 18 months). It contains about one gram of

NUTRIENTS IN 1 TABLESPOON SOY SAUCE*

Calories	11
Protein	1.6 g
Carbohydrate	1.5 g
Vitamin B_2	0.02 mg
Niacin	0.6 mg
Folic acid	2 mg
Pantothenic acid	0.06 mg
Sodium	1029 mg
Potassium	64 mg
Calcium	38 mg
Magnesium	0.49 mg
Phosphorus	38 mg
Zinc	0.04 mg
Copper	0.02 mg

*See Sources, page 103.

protein per four teaspoonsful. It is high in sodium. It does come in a lower-sodium version, but that still may be too high for those on a restricted diet. Also, soy sauce is high in tyramine, a substance that constricts blood vessels and raises blood pressure. If you eat soy sauce while taking antidepressants called MAO inhibitors, it may be difficult for your body to get rid of the tyramine and, as a result, your blood pressure could shoot up.

NUTRIENTS IN 1 TABLESPOON LOWER-SODIUM SOY SAUCE*

Calories	10
Fat	0
Sodium	605 mg
Carbohydrate	1 g
Protein	1 g

*See Sources, page 103.

SOY OIL

Refined soy oil makes up about 75 percent of Americans' vegetable oil intake in various products including cooking oils, mayonnaise, margarine, salad dressings, salad oils, sandwich spreads, vegetable shortening, coffee whiteners,

NUTRIENTS IN 1 TABLESPOON SOY OIL*

	LIQUID	HYDROGENATED
Calories	120	120
Protein	0	0
Total fat	13.6 g	13.6 g
Polyunsaturated fat	2 g	2 g

Cholesterol	0	0
Sodium	Trace	0

*See Sources, page 103.

creamers, and liquid shortening. Soy oil is not associated with the health benefits of most soy products.

SOYBEAN LECITHIN

Lecithin is extracted from soybean oil. It is used commercially as an emulsifying agent in bakery products, candy products, and chocolate coatings. It is, however, of great interest in the medical field. Choline is derived from lecithin. Choline is taken from the digestive tract by the blood and carried to the brain where it becomes acetylcholine, the neurotransmitter that plays a vital part in memory. Possibly because Nature recognized its importance, it is the only neurotransmitter that can be made from another dietary component besides protein. While the exact role and requirement of choline in the diet remains unknown, the brain is unable to make it so choline must be derived from the diet or manufactured in the liver. Researchers are pursuing the idea that the impairment of the brain's system for using choline in certain diseases and in old age may be prevented or minimized by adding choline-based materials to the diet. There has been an effort to increase the building blocks of acetylcholine by increasing lecithin, the normal source of choline in the diet. Purified lecithin, which is more concentrated than that sold in health food stores, raises blood levels of choline, but as yet, there are no definitive studies on the benefits of lecithin.

NUTRIENTS IN 1 TABLESPOON SOYBEAN LECITHIN*

Calories	1204
Protein	0
Total fat	13.6 gm
Polyunsaturated fat	2.1 gm
Fiber	0

*See Sources, page 103.

SOY NUTS

These are roasted, salted soybeans that are crunchy.

NUTRIENTS IN 1 OUNCE SOY NUTS*

Calories	127
Protein	13.3g
Fat	5.5 g
Cholesterol	1 g
Fiber	1 g
Vitamin B$_1$	0.08 mg
Sodium	19 mg
Potassium	336 mg
Calcium	68 mg
Magnesium	1.40 mg

*See Sources, page 103.

MISO

This is a strong, thick, soybean paste made from soybeans, salt, and a fermenting agent, usually an *Aspergillus oryzae* mold culture. Sometimes a grain, such as rice or barley, is added to the mix for additional flavor. The variety of color, flavor, and texture is a reflection of the ingredients and climate in which they were made. Miso soup is a popular appetizer and breakfast drink in Japan. Hacho miso is dark and rich. It is aged a full three years in wooden kegs weighted with stones to allow time, temperature, and climate to create it. Miso has an intense flavor and is used for soups, sauces, dressings, or marinades. It is low in protein and high in sodium. In fact, it can be about 8 to 14 percent salt. A tablespoon of salt has 6589 milligrams of sodium while miso contains 680 milligrams of sodium. There are three basic traditional misos:

- Hacho is made only of soybeans. It is the strongest of the three and is aged as long as three years.
- Mugi is made of soybeans and barley and is milkier. It is aged only about eighteen months.
- Kome is made of soybeans and rice and ages only six months. It is the mildest of the three.

There are infinite varieties of miso, however. Eden-Soy, a company in Clinton, Michigan, produces and sells misos. Their soba miso is made with buckwheat and soybeans, and is a hearty variety that is especially good in cold weather. Since it is a fermented food, miso remains fresh a long time.

On the average, miso contains 12 to 21 percent protein. This compares to chicken, which contains 20 percent protein, and eggs, 13 percent by weight. It also contains helpful enzymes that stimulate digestion.

In Japan, miso is judged and evaluated much like fine wine or cheese in the West. The antioxidant components of miso are being studied as a means of inhibiting the formation of oxidized cholesterol that forms plaque in the arteries. Properly stored, miso can keep for months.

A good source of protein, fiber, and the B vitamins, it also has tyramine, an amino acid that may raise blood pressure, especially if you are taking an MAO inhibitor–type antidepressant, and a very high salt content.

NUTRIENTS IN 2 TABLESPOONS MISO*	
Calories	71
Protein	4 g
Fat	2 g
Carbohydrate	9 g
Calcium	23 mg
Iron	1 mg
Zinc	1.25 mg

*See Sources, page 103.

NATTO

This is fermented, cooked soybeans with a sticky, viscous coating. The Japanese like to use this as a spread or in soups. It is high in protein, rich in fiber, and lower in sodium than miso and soy sauce. It contains iron and other minerals as well as the B vitamins. Remember, though, it is a fermented soy product and contains tyramine, an amino acid that may raise your blood pressure to dangerous levels if you are taking an antidepressant MAO inhibitor.

NUTRIENTS IN ½ CUP NATTO*

Calories	187
from fat	88%
Total fat	9.7 g
Saturated fat	1.4 g
Monounsaturated fat	2.1 g
Polyunsaturated fat	5.5 g
Cholesterol	0
Sodium	6 mg
Protein	15.6 g
Carbohydrate	12.6 g
Fiber	4.8 g
Iron	7.6 mg
Magnesium	101.2 mg
Calcium	191.0 mg
Vitamin C	11.4 mg
Zinc	2.7 mg
Potassium	641.5 mg
Riboflavin	0.2 mg
Thiamine	0.1 mg
Vitamin B$_6$	0.1 mg

*See Sources, page 103.

SOY FLOUR

Developed in the 1940s, this is the simplest form of soy protein. Soybean flour contains practically no starch and is widely used in dietetic foods. The flour is produced by grinding and screening defatted flakes. Defatted soy flakes are the basis of soy protein products. The protein content is about 50 percent. Defatted soy flour adds protein and improves the crust color and shelf life of baked goods. It creates a heavy bread and must be combined with other flours in baking. It may be substituted for some flour in baking, but because it is gluten-free, it cannot replace all the wheat or rye flour in bread recipes. Usually, it can be used as a substitute for up to 20 percent of wheat flour in any recipe. Full-fat flour is made from whole soybeans. This flour contains all the oil, protein, and dietary fiber contained in the whole bean. It is used for doughnut mixes, piecrusts, pancake batters, and other baked goods. Soy flour can become rancid, so store it in the refrigerator or freezer.

NUTRIENTS IN 3½ OUNCES SOY FLOUR*

	FULL-FAT ROASTED	DEFATTED
Calories	441	329
Protein	34.8 g	47 g
Fat	21.9 g	1.2 g
Carbohydrate	33.7 g	38.4 g
Fiber	2.2 g	4.3 g
Calcium	188 mg	241 mg
Iron	5.8 mg	9.2 mg
Zinc	3.5 mg	2.4 mg
Thiamine (B$_1$)	0.41 mg	0.7 mg
Riboflavin	0.94 mg	25 mg
Niacin	3.29 mg	2.61 mg
Magnesium	8.98 mg	11.09 mg

*See Sources, page 103.

SOY POWDER

Soy flour is made by grinding whole dry soybeans into flour in the same way wheat kernels are ground into wheat flour. Soy powder, on the other hand, is made by cooking the soybeans before grinding. It is finer than flour and has less of a beany flavor. It can be used to make soy milk and in baking recipes. It is very easy to use instead of milk powder in coffee and other drinks.

NUTRIENTS IN ¼ CUP SOY POWDER*

	AMOUNT PER SERVING	% DAILY VALUE
Calories	100	
from fat	20	
Total fat	5 g	6% of daily value
Saturated fat	1 g	7% of daily value
Cholesterol	0	0% of daily value
Sodium	1 mg	0% of daily value
Carbohydrate	7 g	2% of daily value
Fiber	3.5g	14% of daily value
Sugars	0 g	0g of daily value
Protein	10 g	Recommended 8 g/kg of weight
Vitamin A	-	0% of daily value
Iron	2.25 mg	15% of daily value
Calcium	144 mg	4% of daily value
Vitamin C	-	0% of daily value

* Daily Values are based on a 2000-calorie diet. Your daily values may be higher or lower depending on your calorie needs.

SOY PROTEIN ISOLATES, CONCENTRATES, AND GRITS

Soy protein isolates from soy flour are highly processed. Developed in the 1950s through a chemical process, most of the protein is withdrawn from defatted soy flakes, resulting in a product with about 90 percent protein content and very little moisture. In fact, the isolates contain the most protein of all soy products, but they have no fiber or carbohydrates. Isolates are used to add texture to meat products and are valued for their emulsifying properties. Soy isolates are the chief component of many dairylike products, including cheese, milk, nondairy frozen desserts, and coffee whiteners. They are in soy hotdogs, soy ice cream, bakery ingredients, noodles, meat products, cereals, prepared mixes, food drinks, baby food, hypoallergenic milk, confections, candy products, special diet foods, and meat analogs.

Soy protein isolates have been used in infant formula in the United States since 1960 for infants that are milk- or lactose- (milk sugar) intolerant. These infant formulas are available in liquid and powder forms. Soy protein isolates are also a protein source in special formulas for older infants, geriatrics, hospitals, and postoperative feeding. Many athletic and health food supplements also contain soy protein isolates.

Soy concentrates, which are produced by the acid removal of carbohydrate from defatted soy flakes, were developed in the 1960s. The remaining concentrated protein may be marketed as a coarse powder, but it is usually textured into flakes, crumbles, or chunks. It is used by institutions to extend meat recipes and commercially to create chicken, veal, or beef patties. *Concentrates* help foods retain moisture. They also add texture and protein. Surimi, protein drinks, and soup bases and gravies contain soy concentrates. These products contain about 70 percent protein while retaining most of the beans' dietary fiber.

Soy grits are a crude form of processed protein. They are made by steam cleaning, hulling, and grinding the beans. They taste like soybeans, have a similar nutritional value, contain 55 to 65 percent protein by weight, and retain most of the original plant components. Grits cook more quickly and are good texturizers for stews, chili, and spaghetti sauces. They are also a good substitute for ground beef because they have a similar texture. You can add them to your chopped meat to extend it and cut down on the fat while benefiting from the soy.

NUTRIENTS IN 1 OUNCE SOY PROTEIN ISOLATES*

Calories	95
Protein	22.60 g
Total fat	0.95 g
Saturated fat	0.15 mg
Polyunsaturated fat	0.61 g
Monounsaturated fat	0.19 g
Carbohydrate	2.10 g
Crude fiber	0.07 g
Calcium	50 mg
Iron	4. mg
Zinc	1.10 mg
Thiamine	0.05 mg
Riboflavin	0.03 mg
Niacin	0.40 mg
Vitamin B_6	n/a
Folacin	49.30 mg

* See Sources, page 103.

TEXTURIZED SOY PROTEIN

Often called texturized vegetable protein (TVP), it is made from soy flour that is compressed to change its texture to a dried, granular product. It is used as an extender in many foods and is the basis for veggie burgers.

NUTRIENTS IN 1 CUP TEXTURIZED SOY PROTEIN (TVP)*

Calories	120
Protein	22 g
Fat	0.2 g
Carbohydrate	14 g
Calcium	170 mg

Iron	4 mg	
Sodium	7 mg	
Zinc	2.7 mg	

* Sources: *Composition of Foods: Legumes and Legume Products,* U.S. Department of Agriculture, Human Nutrition Information Service; Soyfoods Association of America; Rinzler, Carol Ann, *Complete Book of Food* (Mahwah, N.J.: World Almanac, 1987); Pennington, Jean, and Helen Church, *Food Values of Portions Commonly Used* (New York: Harper & Row, 1985); Bricklin, Mark, *Nutrition Advisor* (New York: MJF Books, 1993). The values should be used only as an approximate guide. *Nutrition Labeling* (Washington, D.C.: National Academy Press, 1990).

CONVENIENCE SOY FOODS

The supermarkets and the health food stores are now supplying an increasing choice of convenience soy products. *Environmental Nutrition,* a newsletter of diet, nutrition, and health, has evaluated a number of those foods and the findings are reprinted with permission for your information.

COMPARISON OF CONVENIENCE SOY PRODUCTS*

BRAND	SERVING SIZE	FAT (G)	SATURATED FATS (G)	SOY PROTEIN (G)	CALORIES	SODIUM (MG)	FIBER (G)
BURGERS							
† Boca Burger Vegan Original	2.5 oz	0	0	12	84	227	5
† Natural Touch Vegan Burger	2.75 oz	0	0	N/A**	70	370	3
† Lightlife Lightburger	3.0 oz	1	0	N/A	110	320	N/A
† Morningstar Farms Garden Vege Patty	2.4 oz	4	0.5	N/A	110	350	4
† Green Giant Harvest Burger Original	3.2 oz	4	1.5	18	140	380	5
† Green Giant Harvest Burger—Italian Style	3.2 oz	4.5	1.5	17	140	370	4
Natural Touch Okara Patty	2.3 oz	12	2	N/A	160	360	3
HOT DOGS							
† Lightlife Smart Dogs	1.5 oz	0	0	9	40	170	N/A

BRAND	SERVING SIZE	FAT (G)	SATURATED FATS (G)	SOY PROTEIN (G)	CALORIES	SODIUM (MG)	FIBER (G)
† Yves Veggie Tofu Wieners	1.3 oz	0.5	0	9	57	247	1
Worthington Food Leanies	1.4 oz	6	1.5	N/A	110	330	3
Loma Linda Big Frank	1.8 oz	7	1	N/A	110	240	2
SAUSAGES							
Lightlife Lean Links Breakfast Sausage	2 links (2.5 oz)	6	2	8	120	260	N/A
† Green Giant Breakfast Links	3 links (2.4 oz)	5	0.5	12	110	340	4
† Morningstar Farms Breakfast Links	2 links (1.6 oz)	5	1	N/A	90	340	2
Worthington Foods Prosage Links	2 links (1.6 oz)	9	1.5	N/A	120	290	2
VEGETARIAN ENTRÉES							
Fantastic Foods Mandarin Chow Mein with Tofu	1 cup	5	1	22	330	1,130	5
Fantastic Foods Shells 'n Curry with Tofu	1 cup	6	1	22	440	940	8
† Legume Classic Enchiladas (2)	11 oz	8	N/A	16	270	390	10
† Legume Vegetable Lasagna with Sauce	11 oz	8	N/A	16	240	520	6
Amy's Kitchen Tofu and Vegetable Lasagna	9.5 oz	10	1	N/A	360	500	4
Amy's Kitchen Macaroni and Soy Cheese	7.5 oz	14	1	N/A	360	540	4
Amy's Kitchen Vegetable Pot Pie	7.5 oz	18	11	N/A	360	540	4
Worthington Foods Vegetarian Chicken Pot Pie	8 oz	27	6	N/A	450	1,080	18

* Foods are ranked within each category according to grams of fat, from lowest to highest.

† = EN Picks. (Burger, not dog and sausage picks contain no more than 5 grams of fat and less then 400 milligrams of sodium per serving. Vegetarian entrée picks contain no more than 10 grams of fat and less than 600 milligrams of sodium per serving.)

** N/A = Not available. Reprinted with permission from *Environmental Nutrition*, 52 Riverside Drive, Suite 15-A, New York, New York 10024–6599.

Chapter 8

EASY WAYS TO ADD SOY TO YOUR DIET

No matter how good some food is for you, if it doesn't taste good, you won't eat it. Many food producers have found this out the hard way.

The most popular soy foods in the United States at this writing are tofu, soy milk, soy sauce, miso, and tempeh. But there is a whole new class of manufactured soy foods, which includes such products as tofu hot dogs, tofu ice cream, veggie burgers, tempeh burgers, soy milk yogurt, soy milk cheeses, and soy flour pancake mix.

The immediate hope for increasing our intake of beneficial soy protein in our traditional meat-and-potatoes diet is for soy dishes that taste, look, and feel like meat and potatoes and our other favorite fat-laden foods. During the past ten years, more than 2000 new soy products have made their way into food stores. There are already many meat analogs—meat-free products—made from soy and other ingredients mixed together to form products that look and taste like meat. Such "meats" may be grilled, used in deli-type sandwiches, and added to stews and soups.

As the producers of imitation foods get better at their task, it will become difficult to tell the difference between a juicy meat steak and a juicy soy steak. Take the case of fooled farmers. According to Greg Olwig, the information manager for the American Soybean Association, attendees at an agricultural meeting in St. Louis had eagerly eaten the "beef stroganoff" listed on the menu. They later learned what they had eaten was really made of soy, not beef. "At first people couldn't believe it," Olwig said. "You couldn't tell the difference." Under ordinary circumstances, a stunt like that might irk hungry heartlanders, but this was a meeting of soy farmers and the lunchtime lesson taught them that there is a great future in soy Stroganoff and dairy analogs—products that look and taste like cheese and ice cream.

Barbara Klein and her colleagues at the University of Illinois are conducting studies with postmenopausal women who are given a variety of soy foods to lower their cholesterol. Klein says that recent research at the University of Illinois has shown that soy protein isolates and associated soy plant estrogens are dietary constituents that are effective in decreasing the risk of cardiovascular disease and cancer. The key is developing acceptable soy-based foods for use in a typical diet.

Klein and her colleagues have developed the following products for human studies with isolated soy protein (ISP) (see page 100):

Muffins (5 g ISP per serving)
    Banana muffins
    Blueberry muffins
    Chocolate cherry muffins
    Pineapple muffins

Quick breads (10 g ISP per serving)
    Apricot nut bread
    Pumpkin bread
    Zucchini bread

Yeast breads *(10 g ISP per serving)*
  Italian flatbread
  Pita bread
  Mini loaf bread
  Pretzels

Other *(5 or 10 g ISP per serving)*
  Fruit-flavored bars
  Peanut butter cookies

None of the above are on the market as yet but may be within a year, Klein said, since a number of companies are interested in making these products containing soy.

"Many studies relied on marginally palatable soy products in animal protein-based diets. Subjects found it difficult to comply with long-term protocols using soy ingredients that had distinctive flavors and textures.

"The slow acceptance of many soy-based products is both image-related [soybeans are often used as animal feed] and sensory-related. Flavors and textures unfamiliar to Western palates has deterred many consumers."

She and her colleagues have developed baked goods that are very palatable and they have had good compliance from the women in the study. The muffins have 5 grams of soy protein.

"We want to get them to a point where some companies will be glad to pick them up," she said.

Klein maintains that there are good-tasting soy protein isolates on the market right now, such as Harvest Burgers and a few other health food–type things.

Baked products, she notes, are relatively low in sodium. There are soy milk beverages and a company that produces very concentrated protein isolates.

"We suggest exchanging roughly half the average woman's seventy to ninety grams of protein per day for soy protein," the University of Illinois researcher said. "You could buy the protein powder and mix it in orange juice, milk, or cream-style soup and get yourself up to forty-seven to fifty grams of protein per day."

Klein explained that twenty-five grams of soybean protein is about an ounce of pure powder. She said you could mix the protein powder in your coffee or juice during the day, for example, and easily get up to a therapeutic amount.

The following is a sample of a diet modification plan developed by Klein and her associates at the University of Illinois for an individual using isolated soy protein—supplemented products to provide thirty-five grams of soy protein:

TYPICAL DIET	WITH ISP	MODIFIED WITH ISP PRODUCT
BREAKFAST		
Orange juice, 178 ml	Orange juice, 178 ml	Orange juice, 178 ml, blended with 15 g ISP protein
Bran flakes with skim milk	ISP blueberry muffin (5 g protein)	
Bagel with cream cheese	ISP pita bread (10 g protein)	Banana (whole)
	Banana (half)	
LUNCH		
Vegetable soup	Vegetable soup	Vegetable soup
Tuna salad sandwich on whole wheat bread	Tuna salad sandwich on ISP flatbread (10 g protein)	Tuna salad sandwich on ISP flatbread (10 g protein)
Small candy bar	ISP pumpkin muffin (5 g protein)	ISP pumpkin muffin (5 g protein)
DINNER		
Sirloin steak, 142 g	Sirloin steak, 114 g	Sirloin steak, 86 g
Green beans and onions	ISP bread stick (5 g protein)	Green beans and onions

Steamed potato	Cantaloupe	Cantaloupe
Cantaloupe	Red wine, 178 ml	Red wine, 173 ml
Red wine, 178 ml		
AMOUNT OF SOY PROTEIN 0	AMOUNT OF SOY PROTEIN 35 G	AMOUNT OF SOY PROTEIN 35 G

---

*Reprinted with permission of Barbara Klein and the *Journal of Nutrition: The Official Publication of the American Institute of Nutrition.*

SOME OTHER EASY WAYS TO ADD SOY TO YOUR DIET

So you're a believer in soy's benefits and you want to add more soy to your diet. The recipes on pages 113 through 161 will help you, but you can also add soy without cooking.

- Pour soy milk over breakfast cereal or mix it half-and-half with dairy milk.
- Add soy milk to coffee in place of milk or creamer.
- Puree soft tofu and add it to salad dressings, dips, milkshakes, and cheesecake recipes.
- Use soy milk or part soy milk when making pudding, cream soups, sauces, or pancakes.
- Crumble firm tofu into the cheese for lasagna. Add it to chili or spaghetti sauce.

SENSIBLE SOYBEAN USE

There is no doubt that as the population increases and the information about the health benefits of soybeans grows, the use of soy products will burgeon. And, as with any edible substance that is used by more and more people, certain members of the population will show sensitivity. A food that has served for years as a substitute for many allergenic foods may itself become the offender.

There is also the possibility that with the publicity over the wonders of soybeans, some people will overdo their intake. As with any substance—medication or food—there can be side effects from overindulgence. Soybeans—especially in the raw milk form—may slightly inhibit thyroid hormone. And although they are rich in calcium, the B vitamins, and protein, the beans may also inhibit absorption of some nutrients such as zinc and iron and you have to make sure your diet contains enough of those elements.

Soybeans are also high in tyramine and, as pointed out earlier in the book, if you have high blood pressure or are taking an MAO inhibitor antidepressant, consult your physician or a nutritionist if you are going to increase your intake of soy.

Irvin Liener, Ph.D., of the Department of Biochemistry at the University of Minnesota pointed out at the Arizona meeting on soybeans and health in 1994 that phytic acid has also been considered antinutritional because it interferes with the availability of certain metals such as calcium, magnesium, zinc, and iron. This has raised the possibility that soybean-derived products such as infant formulas and textured vegetable proteins could lead to mineral deficiency in humans. Direct experiments with humans, he said, have produced conflicting results. In the most meaningful study, he said, conducted by the U.S. Department of Agriculture over a period of six months with fifty-two families given meals containing beef extended with soy protein, measurements of zinc and iron were normal when compared with a control group on a self-selected diet.

Soybeans are high in calcium, fiber, protein, and purine and therefore you should certainly check with your physician first before increasing your soy intake if you are on a:

- Low-calcium diet
- Low-fiber diet
- Low-protein diet
- Low-purine (antigout) diet

Soybeans are a bargain for humans and animals on earth. One acre yields forty-three pounds of edible protein in soybean meal fed to animals. That same acre supplies 600 pounds of protein when taken directly as a vegetable protein.

The soybean is indeed a small package packed with health-promoting substances. It is available in more and more varieties, so use your bean and savor soy.

Chapter 9

Recipes

Soy foods can be a wonderful addition to any culinary repertoire. As they have little taste on their own, they readily absorb the flavors imparted by seasonings and the other ingredients in the dish. Proper cooking and seasoning techniques are critical for making soy foods nutritious as well as tasty, because heat and traditional processing such as fermenting, soaking, boiling, and frying help deactivate the trypsin inhibitors or enzyme blockers present in the raw beans.

The following recipes were contributed by a variety of sources. Special thanks is due to the instructors at the Natural Gourmet Cookery School in New York City: Susan Baldassano, Jeri DeLoach Jackson, Melanie Ferreira, Jenny Matthau, and Roberta Atti Robinson. The Soyfoods Association of America and the Soybean Councils of Ohio and Illinois also contributed recipes.

Regarding the nutritional analysis, please note the following:

1. As these recipes are vegetarian, with three exceptions, they contain no cholesterol.
2. To calculate the nutritional components, I have es-

timated in some cases how much flour, oil, or dressing the individual servings may retain after dredging, frying, or dipping.

3. All analysis is per serving. In the case of dressings, sauces, or dips, I have calculated the serving size to be 2 tablespoons.

May these fine foods contribute to your health and well being.

—Annemarie Colbin, recipes editor

Appetizers

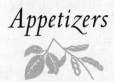

BLACK AND WHITE GARLIC DIP

Serve with crackers or whole wheat pita toasts.

3 garlic cloves, or to taste
¼ cup extra-virgin olive oil
1 pound soft or medium tofu
3 tablespoons fresh lemon juice
¾ teaspoon sea salt, or to taste

¼ cup pitted and sliced Kalamata or other black brine-cured olives
⅛ cup small capers, drained

1. Start the food processor running. Drop the garlic cloves through the processor tube and process until they are finely minced and stuck to the container walls. Stop the processor and scrape the garlic toward the bottom.
2. Add the oil, tofu, lemon juice, and salt and process un-

til very smooth. Taste and adjust the seasonings. Transfer to a bowl.

3. Just before serving, stir in the olives and capers.

Makes about 1 cup

Calories: 108   Protein: 4.7 g   Total fat: 9.78 g   Saturated fat: 1.34 g   Sodium: 251 mg

CHILLED TOFU WITH WATERCRESS, SCALLIONS, AND GINGER

This is a very refreshing dish for hot summer days.

1 pound medium or firm tofu, cut into 1-inch cubes

Ice cubes

½ bunch fresh watercress

1 to 2 carrots, peeled and cut into thin strips with a vegetable peeler

6 scallions, thinly sliced on the diagonal

4 teaspoons grated fresh gingerroot

4 tablespoons dry bonita fish flakes (see Note; optional)

½ cup natural soy sauce (shoyu)

1. Steam the tofu for 2 minutes in a steamer, then transfer to a glass or metal bowl and place in the freezer for 1 hour.

2. Place a few ice cubes in 4 individual bowls, then distribute the tofu cubes on top. Garnish all around each bowl with watercress and carrot strips.

3. Place the sliced scallions, gingerroot, bonita flakes if using, and shoyu in small separate bowls or give each diner individual servings of these garnishes.

4. To eat, dip each tofu cube in the shoyu, put some scallions, ginger, and bonita flakes on top, and enjoy.

Makes 4 servings

Calories: 111   Protein: 10.3 g   Total fat: 5.55 g   Saturated fat: trace   Sodium: 369 mg

Note: Obtainable in Japanese or natural food stores.

CRISPY TEMPEH FINGERS WITH SPICY HONEY-MUSTARD SAUCE

MARINADE

2 cups apple juice

½ cup natural soy sauce (shoyu or tamari)

8 dried shiitake mushrooms

2 whole garlic cloves, peeled

1 tablespoon Dijon mustard

1 teaspoon red pepper flakes

1 (8-ounce) package tempeh, cut crosswise into 12 thin finger-shaped slices

COATING

1 cup cornmeal

½ cup arrowroot or ground kuzu powder

¼ teaspoon salt

Pinch of cayenne

Pinch of ground cumin

¼ cup finely minced fresh parsley

1 cup canola oil for deep frying

DIPPING SAUCE

6 tablespoons honey

3 tablespoons Dijon mustard

2½ tablespoons fresh lemon juice

1½ teaspoons natural soy sauce (shoyu or tamari)

1½ teaspoons cracked red pepper

1 tablespoon chopped fresh dill

Whole radicchio leaves, washed and spun dry

Frisee or red leaf lettuce, washed and spun dry

Parsley sprigs and lemon slices for garnish

1. In a 6-quart pot, mix together the marinade ingredients and bring to a simmer. Add the tempeh and simmer 30 to 40 minutes. Drain.

2. Mix the coating ingredients in a soup or pie plate. Roll each piece of warm tempeh in the coating mixture and place on a cookie sheet or plate; refrigerate for 20 minutes or more.

3. Heat the canola oil in a wok until it is shimmering but not smoking. Fry the tempeh a few pieces at a time until golden brown, then remove with tongs or a slotted spoon and drain on paper towels or brown paper.

4. Combine the dipping sauce ingredients and whisk together. Place in a ramekin.

5. Arrange the radicchio and lettuce leaves on a serving plate and place the ramekin in the center. Arrange the tempeh slices all around. Garnish with parsley sprigs and lemon slices. Serve while warm.

Makes 4 servings

Calories: 281   Protein: 13.1 g   Total fat: 13 g   Saturated fat: 1.37 g   Sodium: 240 mg

Source: *Susan Baldassano, N.Y.*

PHYLLO TRIANGLES WITH SPINACH AND TOFU

1 pound fresh Swiss chard, washed thoroughly

½ pound fresh spinach, washed in several changes of water

1 pound medium-firm or soft tofu

1 tablespoon lemon juice

1 cup packed fresh parsley leaves, chopped

2 tablespoons chopped cilantro (coriander leaf)

½ cup shallots, chopped finely

1 tablespoon extra-virgin olive oil

1 teaspoon sea salt, or to taste

Freshly ground pepper to taste

½ pound (2 sticks) unsalted butter

½ pound phyllo dough

1. Preheat the oven to 425°F.

2. After washing the chard, cut away most of the white stems and place the wet leaves in a pot with the wet washed spinach; cook, covered, over medium heat for 3 to 4 minutes, or until the greens have wilted. Drain and chop fine.

3. Mash the tofu in a large bowl with a fork; add the lemon juice, parsley, and cilantro.

4. In a sauté pan, sauté the shallots in the olive oil until soft, about 3 minutes. Add the cooked chopped greens, salt, and pepper and cook for 2 to 3 minutes, uncovered, to evaporate most of the liquids. Add the greens mixture to the tofu and stir well to blend. Taste and adjust the seasonings. Set aside.

5. Melt the butter over low heat. Unroll the phyllo carefully, cut lengthwise into 3 equal sections, and cover with a damp towel.

6. Remove 1 strip of phyllo onto a flat surface, replacing the damp towel immediately. Brush the phyllo strip with melted butter. Place another strip on top and butter it as well. Place 2 large tablespoonfuls of the greens-tofu mix-

ture in the lower left corner of the buttered phyllo strips; fold the bottom over the filling to align the lower edge with the right side edge, forming a triangle. Continue folding over and over to the top of the pastry strip. Brush with melted butter and place on a cookie sheet lined with parchment paper. Repeat with the rest of the phyllo strips and filling.

7. Bake for 20 to 25 minutes, or until the phyllo is crisp and golden brown. Serve warm.

Makes about 30 pieces (15 servings)

Calories: 165   Protein: 5.28 g   Total fat: 9.98 g   Saturated fat: 4.97 g   Sodium: 224 mg

Soups

CREAMY TOMATO SOUP

2 red onions, diced

4 garlic cloves, minced

½ teaspoon sea salt

2 teaspoons olive oil

3 pounds ripe tomatoes

12 ounces soft or silken tofu

½ cup smooth peanut butter

Dill or parsley sprig for garnish

1. In a large soup pot, sauté the onions and garlic with the salt in the olive oil for 2 minutes over medium-low heat.

2. Cut the tomatoes across the middle; squeeze out the seeds and discard them, then cut the tomatoes in chunks.

Add to the onions, stir, cover, and simmer until the tomatoes are soft and have released a lot of water, about 30 to 45 minutes.

3. Process in batches in a blender or food processor, adding the tofu and peanut butter gradually, until smooth and creamy. Reheat slightly before serving if necessary, but do not boil. Garnish with a sprig of dill or parsley.

Makes 6 servings

Calories: 275   Protein: 12.4 g   Total fat: 15 g   Saturated fat: 3.17 g   Sodium: 207 mg

Source: *Roberta Atti Robinson, N.J.*

THE EASIEST CREAM OF ZUCCHINI SOUP

2 tablespoons extra-virgin olive oil

About 8 cups zucchini and/or yellow squash, cut in large chunks

4 to 5 tablespoons sweet mellow miso, or to taste

Parsley for garnish

1. In a 4-quart heavy-bottomed pot, heat the oil slightly over low heat and add all the zucchini and/or yellow squash. Stir until the squash have started to release some liquid. Cover, keep the heat very low, and allow the vegetables to sweat and release all their liquid. This will take about 30 to 45 minutes. Stir often to prevent burning.

2. The zucchini should have released enough water to be almost covered. Process with the miso, in batches if necessary, in a blender or food processor until smooth and vel-

vety; adjust to your taste with some extra miso if desired.
Garnish with parsley and serve hot or cold.

Makes about 6 servings

**Calories: 83   Protein: 3.2 g   Total fat: 5.26 g   Saturated fat: trace
Sodium: 317 mg**

Source: *Roberta Atti Robinson, N.J.*

ROOT VEGETABLE STEW WITH
TOFU NUGGETS

½ pound firm tofu

2½ quarts water

1 (2-inch) strip of kombu
seaweed

6 dried shiitake mushrooms

1 (½-inch) piece of fresh
gingerroot

1 tablespoon canola oil, plus 2
cups for deep frying

1 onion, diced medium

1 tablespoon minced garlic

1 (6-inch) piece of burdock,
medium roll-cut (optional)

1 large carrot, medium roll-cut

1 small rutabaga (yellow
turnip), peeled and cut into
¾-inch cubes

1 small white turnip, diced
into ¾-inch cubes

1 tablespoon toasted sesame
oil

1 (6-inch) daikon radish,
medium roll-cut

1 small butternut squash,
peeled, seeds removed, and cut
into ¾-inch cubes

¼ cup natural soy sauce (shoyu
or tamari)

1 (2-inch) piece of gingerroot
blended with ¼ cup water,
strained, juice reserved

1 tablespoon mirin (sweet rice
wine) or sherry

¼ cup thinly sliced scallions for
garnish

1. Press the tofu in a bowl or plate under weighted objects
for 30 minutes to remove the water. When ready, cube
small and set aside.

2. Place the water, kombu, mushrooms, and peeled ginger

in a 6-quart pot. Simmer, covered, for 30 to 40 minutes; remove the mushrooms and kombu, slice thin, removing the stems from the mushrooms, and return to the stock. Discard the ginger.

3. Heat 1 tablespoon canola oil over medium heat in a large skillet. Add the onion, garlic, burdock (if using), carrot, rutabaga, and turnip in that order, sautéing a few minutes after each addition. Add the toasted sesame oil, mix well, then add the whole vegetable mixture to the stock.

4. Add the daikon and butternut squash to the stock as well and continue to simmer until the vegetables are very tender, about 20 to 30 minutes.

5. Heat 2 cups canola oil in a wok until it shimmers but does not smoke. When the oil is very hot, deep-fry the tofu cubes until golden brown and place on paper towels or brown paper to drain. Add to the soup.

6. Season the soup with soy sauce, ginger juice, and mirin, adjusting to your taste. Garnish with fresh scallions.

Makes about 8 servings

Calories: 151   Protein: 4.93 g   Total fat: 6.75 g   Saturated fat: trace   Sodium: 551 mg

Source: *Susan Baldassano, N.Y.*

RYOKAN MISO SOUP

5 cups vegetable stock or water

1 (about 1 × 4-inch) strip kombu seaweed

1 ounce bonita fish flakes (optional)

3 large dry shiitake mushrooms, soaked and sliced

2 strips of wakame seaweed, soaked and chopped

½ pound firm tofu, cubed small

3 to 4 tablespoons mellow yellow miso, or to taste

2 scallions, thinly sliced on the diagonal

1. Bring the stock or water to a boil, add the kombu, and simmer 20 minutes. Add the bonita flakes if using and turn the heat off immediately; cover the pot and let the stock sit for about 3 minutes, or until the bonita flakes have fallen to the bottom. Strain out the kombu and flakes.

2. Add the sliced mushrooms and chopped wakame to the stock and bring to a boil. Simmer 5 to 10 minutes. Add the tofu and simmer another 2 minutes.

3. Remove the soup from the heat. Add the miso by mashing it through a strainer. (Do not boil the miso, as it destroys valuable enzymes.) Cover and let sit 2 to 3 minutes. Garnish each bowl with 1 teaspoon scallions.

Makes 4 servings

Calories: 79.6 Protein: 6.27 g   Total fat: 3.4 g   Saturated fat: trace   Sodium: 358 mg

Source: *Melanie Ferreira, N.Y.*

TARRAGON-SCENTED SHIITAKE AND BROCCOLI SOUP WITH TOFU

1 quart chicken or vegetable stock

4 garlic cloves, minced

6 large fresh shiitake mushrooms, thinly sliced, stems removed

4 ounces firm tofu, cubed small

¼ teaspoon crumbled dried tarragon

Pinch of dried ground sage

1 cup broccoli, separated into very small florets

Salt and pepper to taste

Snipped fresh chives for garnish

1. Place the stock, garlic, mushrooms, tofu, and herbs in a 3-quart saucepan. Bring to a boil, lower the heat, cover, and simmer for 15 minutes.

2. Add the broccoli and simmer another 6 to 7 minutes. Taste and adjust the seasonings. Serve hot, garnished with snipped chives.

Makes 6 servings

Calories: 31.3   Protein: 2.4 g   Total fat: 1 g   Saturated fat: trace
Sodium: 189 mg

MINESTRONE WITH TEMPEH AND FRESH HERBS

1 medium onion, chopped

2 garlic cloves, minced

3 tablespoons extra-virgin olive oil

2 teaspoons sea salt, or to taste

8 ounces tempeh, cut in 1-inch cubes

1 large carrot, cut in quarter moons

2 celery stalks, diced (include leaves if organically grown)

1 potato, peeled and diced

1 zucchini, diced

1 large ripe tomato, seeded and chopped

8 cups water or stock

2 tablespoons fresh thyme, chopped

2 tablespoons fresh marjoram, chopped

4 leaves fresh sage, chopped

Chopped parsley or cilantro for garnish

Freshly ground pepper

1. In a 4-quart heavy pot, sauté the onions and garlic in the oil with the salt and tempeh until the onions are wilted, about 3 to 4 minutes.

2. Add the carrot, celery, potato, zucchini, and tomato and continue to sauté for 5 minutes more. Then add the water or stock, bring to a boil, and simmer, covered, for about 30 minutes.

3. Five minutes before the end of the cooking, add the thyme, marjoram, and sage and cook the remaining 5 minutes. Adjust the seasonings, garnish with parsley or cilantro, and serve with a few grinds of pepper.

Makes 8 servings

Calories: 127   Protein: 7 g   Total fat: 7 g   Saturated fat: trace
Sodium: 570 mg

Source: *Roberta Atti Robinson, N.J.*

Salads

CHICORY SALAD WITH CREAMY SESAME DRESSING

1 head chicory, washed, dried, and torn into bite-size pieces

1 cup cooked chickpeas

1 cup thinly sliced red onion

½ cup tahini (sesame paste)

3 tablespoons white or light barley miso

⅓ cup brown rice or apple cider vinegar

2 tablespoons prepared grainy mustard

About ⅓ cup water, or as needed

1 tablespoon toasted sesame seeds

1. Place the chicory in a large salad bowl. Scatter the chickpeas over it, then top with the red onions.
2. In a small bowl, gently mix the tahini with the miso, then blend in the vinegar and mustard. The mixture should

be creamy with no lumps. Thin out further with the water to the desired consistency. Pour over the salad and top with the toasted sesame seeds. Serve immediately.

Makes 6 servings

Calories: 230   Protein: 9.5 g   Total fat: 13.7 g   Saturated fat: 2 g
Sodium: 339 mg

CONFETTI COLESLAW

½ small green cabbage, shredded (about 2 cups)

½ small red cabbage, shredded (about 2 cups)

½ carrot, diced small

1 celery stalk, diced small

2 tablespoons diced fennel stalks

¼ cup diced red pepper

2 tablespoons diced green pepper

½ cup raisins

½ tablespoon caraway seeds, roasted in a 350°F oven for 2 minutes

DRESSING

½ pound silken tofu

¼ cup soy milk

2 tablespoons mustard

2 tablespoons apple cider vinegar

1 tablespoon lemon juice

3 tablespoons honey

1½ teaspoons salt

1 bunch dill, minced (about ⅓ cup)

Freshly ground black pepper to taste

1. Place the cabbages, carrot, celery, fennel, peppers, and raisins in a large bowl and mix well. Add the roasted caraway seeds.
2. Place the dressing ingredients, except for the dill and

pepper, in a food processor or blender and process until smooth and creamy. Add the dill and blend 2 to 3 seconds more. Season with fresh pepper.

3. Fold the dressing into the vegetables and let sit 30 minutes. Toss before serving. Serve over a bed of lettuce.

Makes 6 to 8 servings

Calories: 62   Protein: 1.4 g   Total fat: 3 g   Saturated fat: 0
Sodium: 25.7 mg

Dressing Calories: 47   Protein: 2.2 g   Total fat: 1.3 g   Saturated fat: trace   Sodium: 452 mg

Source: *Susan Baldassano, N.Y.*

CREAMY CAESAR SALAD WITH SUN-DRIED TOMATOES

½ tablespoon minced garlic

½ tablespoon olive oil

½ sheet nori seaweed

½ pound silken tofu

1½ tablespoons white, yellow, or chickpea miso

1½ tablespoons Dijon mustard

3 tablespoons umeboshi (pickled plum) paste (see Note)

¼ cup soy milk

3 sun-dried tomatoes soaked in warm water 20 minutes, drained and minced

2 tablespoons minced fresh parsley

18 ounces (6 big handfuls) mesclun salad or other mixed greens

1. Sauté the garlic in the oil 15 seconds, or until just golden. Set aside.

2. Toast the nori over an open flame for 1 second on each side until it turns a brighter green. With scissors, cut the nori into small ⅛-inch pieces.

3. Place the garlic, tofu, miso, mustard, umeboshi paste, and soy milk in a food processor and process until creamy.

Add the tomatoes, nori, and parsley and blend another 2 to 3 seconds. Toss with the greens and serve immediately.

Makes 6 to 8 servings

Calories: 52   Protein: 3.8 g   Total fat: 2.5 g   Saturated fat: trace
Sodium: 251 mg

Source: *Susan Baldassano, N.Y.*

Note: Obtainable in health food stores.

MINTED PASTA AND TOFU SALAD

1 cup French lentils, soaked overnight and drained

1 teaspoon sea salt

½ pound small pasta, like orzo, fusilli, or small shells, whole wheat if available

2 plum tomatoes, seeded and chopped

1 cucumber, peeled, seeded, and diced

¼ cup loosely packed mint leaves, chopped

3 scallions, whites and greens, chopped

1 yellow bell pepper, seeded and diced

1 small red onion, diced

4 to 6 fresh basil leaves, chopped

6 radicchio leaves

6 ounces arugula

DRESSING

2½ tablespoons balsamic vinegar

5 tablespoons extra-virgin olive oil

2½ tablespoons lemon juice

1 teaspoon sea salt

2 garlic cloves, pressed

½ pound extra-firm tofu, diced

Soy sauce, if needed

Freshly ground black pepper to taste

1. Cook the lentils in 4 cups water with the salt until soft but still whole, about 40 minutes. Drain and set aside.

Cook the pasta until it is *al dente*. Drain and submerge in cold water until ready to use.

2. Prepare the vegetables and herbs. Drain the pasta well and combine with the lentils, tomatoes, cucumber, mint, scallions, pepper, onion, and basil.

3. Combine all the dressing ingredients in a separate bowl, whisking till emulsified, and add to the pasta. Toss gently. Add the tofu and toss again. If desired, sprinkle a little soy sauce over all. Serve on a bed of radicchio and arugula and season with pepper.

Makes 6 servings

Calories: 148   Protein: 9 g   Total fat: 2 g   Saturated fat: trace
Sodium: 123 mg

Dressing Calories: 103   Protein: trace   Total fat: 11 g   Saturated fat: 1.5 g   Sodium: 356 mg

Source: *Roberta Atti Robinson, N.J.*

MIXED GREENS VINAIGRETTE WITH TEMPEH CROUTONS

¼ *pound (½ package) Seasoned Tempeh (page 137) (see Note)*

2 *cups canola oil for deep-frying*

DRESSING

1½ *tablespoons white balsamic vinegar or 1 tablespoon dark balsamic vinegar*

4½ *tablespoons extra-virgin olive oil*

1 *tablespoon Dijon mustard*

½ *cup fresh parsley, minced*

¼ *teaspoon salt*

¾ *pound (4 big handfuls) mesclun salad or baby greens, washed and spun dry*

1 *large tomato, cut into thin wedges*

1. Cut the seasoned tempeh into ¼-inch cubes.

2. Heat the canola oil in a wok until it shimmers but does not smoke. With a slotted spoon, add the tempeh a few pieces at a time. When they turn golden brown, remove and set on paper towels or brown paper to drain.

3. In a small bowl, whisk the vinegar, mustard, and salt together; then add the oil in a steady stream to emulsify. Alternatively, duplicate the procedure in a blender, pouring the oil slowly through the top while the motor is running. Stir in the parsley at the end.

4. Combine the mesclun and tomatoes. Add enough dressing to moisten and garnish with the tempeh croutons.

Makes 4 to 6 servings

Calories: 142   Protein: 5 g   Total fat: 12 g   Saturated fat: 1.5 g   Sodium: 196 mg

Source: *Susan Baldassano, N.Y.*

Note: See Crispy Tempeh Fingers with Spicy Honey-Mustard Sauce, page 115, for a different marinade for the tempeh.

Main Dishes / Entrées

BAKED BEANS WITH MISO AND APPLE BUTTER

2 cups dried kidney beans, soaked and drained

6 cups water

1½ teaspoons Pommery or other whole grain mustard

1 tablespoon grated onion

1½ tablespoons mellow barley or brown rice miso

| ¼ cup unsweetened unspiced apple butter | 2 teaspoons brown rice or apple cider vinegar |

1. Place the beans and water in a 3-quart saucepan and cook, covered, over low heat until tender, about 45 minutes. Drain, reserving 1 cup cooking liquid.
2. Preheat the oven to 350°F. In a bowl, mix the miso, apple butter, mustard, onion, vinegar, and reserved bean cooking liquid. Add the beans and mix gently.
3. Place the beans in a heavy, oiled 3-quart covered casserole, cover, and bake for 1½ hours. Serve hot.

Makes 6 servings

Calories: 238   Protein: 14 g   Total fat: 1 g   Saturated fat: trace
Sodium: 164 mg

BROCCOLI, WILD MUSHROOM, AND TOFU QUICHE

This is good for lunch with a soup and salad.

6 ounces fresh wild mushrooms (shiitake, oyster, chanterelle, or porcini), sliced, stems removed

6 ounces white button mushrooms, wiped clean and thinly sliced

1 prepared unsweetened piecrust

2 teaspoons extra-virgin olive oil

4 garlic cloves, minced

1 teaspoon sea salt, or to taste

1 teaspoon dried basil

1 teaspoon dried marjoram

1 cup very small broccoli florets

1½ pounds soft tofu

2 tablespoons lemon juice

2 tablespoons cold-pressed sunflower oil

Freshly ground black pepper to taste

1. Preheat the oven to 350°F. Prepare the vegetables.
2. Prebake the crust for 6 to 7 minutes, or until it sounds slightly hollow when tapped.
3. In a large skillet, heat the oil and sauté the garlic for 15 seconds, then add the mushrooms and ¼ teaspoon sea salt. Lower the heat and continue stirring for 4 to 5 minutes. Sprinkle on the basil and marjoram and cook another 2 to 3 minutes, until most of the mushroom liquid has evaporated.
4. Boil 1 quart of water and blanch the broccoli florets in it for 15 seconds, or just until they turn a bright green. Drain and plunge briefly into a bowl of cold water to stop the cooking. Drain and set aside.
5. Place the tofu, lemon juice, remaining ¾ teaspoon salt, and sunflower oil in a blender or food processor and blend until very smooth and creamy. It should be the consistency of thick but pourable sour cream. If too thick, add 1 tablespoon water.
6. Assemble the quiche. Spread the mushrooms over the bottom of the prebaked crust, top with the broccoli florets, grind some fresh pepper over them, then top with the creamed tofu, smoothing it over with a spatula and making sure the vegetables are completely covered. Bake for 30 minutes, or until the ridges of the tofu take on a beige hue. Serve hot or cold.

Makes 6 to 8 servings

Calories: 233   Protein: 8 g   Total fat: 15 g   Saturated fat: 3 g
Sodium: 413 mg

CALICO CHILI

1½ cups dried edible soybeans, soaked overnight

1 cup chopped carrots

⅓ cup each chopped red, green, and yellow bell peppers

1 cup chopped onions

1 cup chopped celery

3 garlic cloves, minced

2 (16-ounce) cans chili-style diced tomatoes

1 (16-ounce) can dark red kidney beans, drained

2 tablespoons chili con carne seasoning

2 tablespoons seasoned pepper

1 teaspoon dried oregano

CONDIMENTS

Any kind of low-fat or regular shredded cheese (e.g., Monterrey Jack, cheddar)

Chopped fresh cilantro

Chopped onions

1. Place dry beans in 6 cups water and soak overnight. Remove and drain.

2. Place soybeans in a pot with 4 cups water, bring to a boil, and simmer, covered, for 1 hour. Drain. Place the beans, carrots, peppers, onions, celery, garlic, tomatoes, kidney beans, and seasonings in a Crock-Pot. Stir well to blend. Set on low and cook for 8 to 10 hours. Top with the condiments as desired.

Makes 8 to 10 servings

Calories: 159 Protein: 9 g   Total fat: 4 g   Saturated fat: trace
Sodium: 462 mg

Source: *Ohio Soybean Council*

FAMILY-STYLE BEAN CURD

1 block firm tofu (about 1 pound)

2 cups safflower or canola oil for deep-frying

1⅓ cups stock or water

2 tablespoons natural soy sauce (shoyu or tamari)

½ tablespoon ginger juice (see Note)

2 tablespoons dark or hot
sesame oil

6 scallions, whites and greens
separated and cut into 2-inch
pieces

½ tablespoon minced fresh
gingerroot

3 large dried shiitake mushrooms soaked in 2 cups water
for ½ hour

½ cup sliced bamboo shoots
(optional)

1 tablespoon sweet rice wine or
sherry

1 tablespoon arrowroot or
kuzu powder

1 tablespoon cold water

1. Cut the tofu into triangles or large cubes. Heat the oil in a wok or medium skillet, add the tofu, and deep-fry on both sides until golden brown, about 3 to 4 minutes. Drain on brown paper or paper towels. Pour the oil out of the wok and discard.*

2. Simmer the deep-fried tofu in a small pan with the stock or water, soy sauce, and ginger juice for about 8 to 10 minutes. Drain and reserve 1 cup of the liquid.

3. Heat the wok and add the sesame oil. Stir-fry the scallion whites and minced gingerroot for 1 minute. Add the mushrooms, bamboo shoots if using, and scallion greens and stir a few times. Then add the seasoned tofu, 1 cup tofu cooking liquid, and rice wine or sherry. Simmer 3 minutes.

4. Dissolve the arrowroot or kuzu in the cold water and add, stirring continuously until the sauce thickens. Serve hot over rice or noodles.

Makes 4 to 6 servings

Calories: 142   Protein: 7 g   Total fat: 10.5 g   Saturated fat: 1.3 g
Sodium: 352 mg

Note: To make ginger juice, grate 2 to 3 inches of ginger—no need to peel—and squeeze the gratings by hand, in a cheesecloth, or in a garlic press to obtain the ginger juice.

Source: *Melanie Ferreira, N.Y.*

* Add detergent and water to the used oil before pouring it down the drain.

MARINATED TOFU KABOBS

MARINADE

¼ cup apple cider vinegar

2 tablespoons soy sauce

2 scallions, chopped

1 teaspoon grated gingerroot

¼ cup frozen orange juice concentrate

2 tablespoons lemon juice

KABOBS

8 pearl onions, peeled

8 medium button mushrooms

8 small whole potatoes, cooked

16 (1-inch-square) pieces of green pepper

1 pound firm tofu, cut into 1-inch cubes

8 cherry tomatoes

1. Mix the marinade ingredients together.
2. Place the onions, mushrooms, potatoes, green pepper, and tofu cubes in a large resealable plastic bag and set the bag in a large bowl. Pour the marinade over the vegetables and close the bag. Marinate for 4 hours in the refrigerator, turning the bag several times.
3. Thread the marinated ingredients, along with the cherry tomatoes, alternately on 4 skewers. Place on a broiler rack or outdoor grill. Cook about 8 minutes, turning once and basting several times with the marinade.

Makes 4 servings

Calories: 239   Protein: 13 g   Total fat: 7 g   Saturated fat: trace
Sodium: 447 mg

Source: *United Soybean Board, Ill.*

NICKY'S RICE AND TEMPEH SPECIALTY

8 ounces tempeh, boiled in water to cover for 10 minutes and cut in small dice

2 tablespoons canola oil

3 tablespoons natural soy sauce (shoyu or tamari)

2 cups washed and tightly packed raw spinach

4 cups cooked brown rice

1 cup toasted sesame seeds

1. In a skillet, sauté the tempeh in the oil and soy sauce over low heat, until golden brown. Set aside.
2. Cook the washed spinach by placing it in a saucepan on a low flame, covered (the water remaining on it will be sufficient for steaming), for 5 minutes. Then strain it and squeeze out the excess water. Chop very finely.
3. Add the tempeh and spinach to the rice, mix well, and form little rice balls of about 2-inch diameter. Roll the rice balls in the sesame seeds and serve as a side dish or snack.

Makes 8 servings

Calories: 402   Protein: 18 g   Total fat: 15 g   Saturated fat: 2.5 g
Sodium: 570 mg

Source: *Roberta Atti Robinson, N.J.*

SPAGHETTI AGLIO E OLIO WITH TEMPEH CROSTINI

½ cup extra-virgin olive oil

6 garlic cloves, sliced

1 or 2 dry hot red peppers

MARINADE

1 cup water

3 tablespoons umeboshi vinegar

8 ounces tempeh, cut in half lengthwise and then in ¼-inch slices

Canola oil for panfrying

1 pound spaghetti or linguine

3 garlic cloves, pressed

1 sprig of fresh rosemary or 1 tablespoon dried

2 tablespoons salt for pasta cooking water

1 bunch parsley (about 1½ cups loosely packed), chopped

1 pint oil-cured black olives, pitted and chopped

1. Heat the oil with the sliced garlic and peppers, making sure the garlic does not burn, for about 1 minute. Remove from the heat and let the oil cool. Discard the garlic and peppers and set the oil aside.

2. Combine the marinade ingredients in a 2-quart saucepan and bring to a simmer. Add the tempeh slices, and simmer for 10 minutes. Strain the tempeh, pat dry with paper towels, then panfry in canola oil on both sides until golden and crispy. Set aside. (The marinade can be used for flavoring another dish.)

3. Cook the pasta until al dente in the salted water. Strain and toss with the flavored oil, parsley, and olives. Top with the tempeh crostini and serve immediately.

Makes 8 servings

Calories: 221   Protein: 9 g   Total fat: 12 g   Saturated fat: 1.5 g
Sodium: 188 mg

Source: *Roberta Atti Robinson, N.J.*

SEASONED TEMPEH

Tempeh needs good seasoning to be made appetizing. The following is a recipe that can be used as a standard in many dishes.

1 (8-ounce) package tempeh

1¾ cups water

2 garlic cloves, smashed flat

¼ cup natural soy sauce (shoyu or tamari)

3 slices fresh gingerroot

Slice the tempeh into the desired shape—cubes, fingers, or rectangles—or leave whole. Place in a 3-quart pot with the rest of the ingredients. Simmer, covered, for 10 minutes. Drain in a colander; reserve the cooking liquid if required in recipes, discarding the garlic and ginger. Do not reuse the cooking liquid for another batch of tempeh. Increase the quantities exactly for larger amounts of tempeh. The seasoned tempeh can be frozen for later use.

Makes 4 servings

Calories: 94   Protein: 12.4 g   Total fat: 3 g   Saturated fat: trace
Sodium: 264 mg

Note: 1 teaspoon cumin and 1 teaspoon curry powder can be used instead of ginger and garlic.

SPROUTED BEANS AND TOFU CURRY

1 pound extra-firm tofu

1 cup assorted sprouted beans (lentils, peas, garbanzo, adzuki, mung, or the like)

1 small or medium onion, diced (about ¾ cup)

2 tablespoons extra-virgin olive oil

2 sweet potatoes (yams), peeled and diced medium

½ teaspoon ground cardamom

½ teaspoon celery seeds

½ teaspoon paprika

½ to 1 teaspoon curry powder

1 large ripe red or yellow tomato

1 cup water

½ teaspoon sea salt or vegetable salt

2 tablespoons canola oil

2 tablespoons Worcestershire sauce or natural soy sauce (shoyu or tamari)

Chopped fresh mint for garnish

1. Place a salad plate upside down in a bowl, place the tofu on top, and place another plate on top of the tofu to press out the water. For added weight, place a pint container with beans or water on the top plate. Let sit for 30 minutes. Discard the water and cut the tofu into 1-inch cubes.

2. Simmer the sprouted beans in water to cover (about 2½ or 3 cups) for about 20 minutes, or until soft.

3. In a heavy 4-quart pot, sauté the onions in the olive oil for 2 minutes, then add the sweet potatoes, cardamom, celery seeds, paprika, curry powder, tomato, water, and salt. Cover and simmer over low heat for about 10 minutes.

4. In a skillet, heat the canola oil. Add the tofu and Worcestershire sauce; brown the tofu lightly. Add to the onion mixture together with the cooked beans with their water. Stir and continue to cook for another 10 minutes. Serve hot on top of rice, noodles, or a grain of your choice, garnished with fresh mint.

Makes about 6 servings

Calories: 222   Protein: 9 g   Total fat: 13 g   Saturated fat: 1.5 g
Sodium: 542 mg

Source: *Roberta Atti Robinson, N.J.*

TEMPEH SCALOPPINE

4 cups water

¼ cup natural soy sauce (shoyu or tamari)

4 slices of fresh gingerroot

1 strip of kombu seaweed (about 4 inches)

1 teaspoon sea salt

1 (8-ounce) package tempeh

2 cups unbleached white flour

3 tablespoons olive oil

1 cup tempeh cooking liquid

½ cup stock or water

4 fresh lemon wedges

Sprigs of fresh thyme for garnish

1. In a medium saucepan, combine the water, soy sauce, ginger slices, kombu, and sea salt. Heat, add the whole tempeh block, and simmer, covered, for 20 minutes. To keep the tempeh under the liquid, place a small plate or heat-resistant bowl on top while it simmers. The tempeh will turn a light, golden brown color when done. Remove and reserve 1 cup liquid.

2. Cut the tempeh block in half horizontally, then vertically on the diagonal to make pieces about 2 × 2 inches. Dredge them in the flour and place on a clean plate.

3. Heat the oil in a large skillet and fry the tempeh on both sides for 2 to 3 minutes. Add the tempeh cooking liquid and stock, cover, and bring to a boil. Stir once. Simmer 5 to 6 minutes, uncover, and keep cooking until the liquid reduces somewhat and is thickened by the flour to a saucelike consistency. Serve immediately over cooked fettuccine or rice, garnishing with a lemon wedge and thyme sprigs.

Makes 2 to 4 servings

**Calories: 236   Protein: 14 g   Total fat: 13 g   Saturated fat: 2 g
Sodium: 399 mg**

Source: *Melanie Ferreira, N.Y.*

TEMPEH WITH SWEET-AND-SOUR SAUCE

2 tablespoons vegetable oil

1 recipe Seasoned Tempeh (page 137), cut into cubes

1 cup unfiltered apple juice

½ cup reserved tempeh cooking liquid

2 tablespoons lemon juice

½ teaspoon sea salt

2 tablespoons apple cider vinegar

¼ cup maple syrup

1 tablespoon prepared whole grain mustard

3 tablespoons kuzu or arrowroot powder

Grated rind from ½ orange, preferably organically grown

1. In a large skillet, heat the oil and sauté the tempeh over high heat until lightly browned. Set aside.

2. In a 2-quart saucepan, combine ½ cup apple juice, the tempeh broth, lemon juice, salt, vinegar, maple syrup, and mustard. Heat.

3. Dissolve the kuzu or arrowroot powder in the remaining ½ cup apple juice and add the orange rind. Add to the saucepan, stirring until the mixture has thickened. Add the tempeh cubes, mix, and serve over rice or pasta.

Makes 4 servings

Calories: 261   Protein: 13 g   Total fat: 10 g   Saturated fat: 1 g
Sodium: 841 mg

TEMPEH WITH SHALLOTS AND WHITE WINE

1 recipe Seasoned Tempeh (page 137)

½ cup whole wheat pastry flour

3 tablespoons olive oil

2 garlic cloves, minced

3 shallots, minced

½ cup dry white wine

2 tablespoons reserved tempeh
cooking liquid

3 tablespoons water

1 teaspoon fresh lemon juice

1 tablespoon chopped fresh
parsley

1. When making the seasoned tempeh, slice it horizontally through the middle into 2 layers, then cut vertically into 8 rectangles.

2. Place the flour in a soup plate or pie plate and roll the moist seasoned tempeh in it to cover. Set the floured tempeh on a separate plate.

3. In a large skillet or sauté pan, heat 1 tablespoon olive oil and add the garlic and shallots. Sauté for 2 to 3 minutes over medium heat, or until translucent. Set aside in a bowl or on a small plate.

4. Add the rest of the oil to the same skillet and heat. Add the floured tempeh and panfry several minutes on each side, until lightly browned. Add the reserved garlic and shallots.

5. Add the wine to deglaze the pan, then the reserved tempeh liquid, water, and lemon juice. Stir well and cook over medium heat for about 15 minutes, until the liquids have reduced to half and thickened from the flour. Serve hot with rice and steamed vegetables, garnished with the chopped parsley.

Makes 4 servings

Calories: 251   Protein: 14 g   Total fat: 13 g   Saturated fat: 2 g
Sodium: 345 mg

TOFU MUSHROOM STROGANOFF

1 pound green beans, trimmed and snapped into 2-inch pieces

¾ cup water

2 cups chopped onions

2 tablespoons canola or sunflower oil

1 red pepper, seeded and chopped

12 ounces white mushrooms, chopped

¼ teaspoon sea salt

3 tablespoons whole wheat pastry flour

3 tablespoons natural soy sauce (shoyu or tamari)

Freshly ground pepper

TOFU SOUR CREAM

1 pound soft tofu

3 tablespoons canola or sunflower oil

2½ tablespoons fresh lemon juice (about 1 large lemon)

2 scallions, white part only, chopped

1 teaspoon brown rice vinegar

½ teaspoon sea salt

1½ tablespoons chopped fresh dill

1. In a small saucepan, steam the green beans with the water for 5 minutes. Drain and set aside, reserving the liquid.
2. In a skillet, sauté the onions in the oil until soft, about 3 to 4 minutes. Add the red pepper and mushrooms; sprinkle the sea salt over them. Cook, stirring, until the mushrooms release their liquid, about 3 to 4 minutes. Sprinkle the flour over all, stir, and continue cooking a few minutes more, until the flour has absorbed all the liquid.
3. Add the green bean cooking water a little at a time, stirring constantly to blend well. Simmer, covered, for 15 minutes, until thickened, stirring occasionally. Add the soy sauce and fresh pepper and simmer another 5 minutes.
4. To make the tofu sour cream, combine the tofu, oil, lemon juice, scallions, brown rice vinegar, and salt in a

blender or food processor and process until smooth and creamy.

5. Stir the tofu sour cream into the onion mixture, then add the green beans and heat briefly. Adjust the seasonings. Add the chopped dill and serve immediately over hot udon noodles, linguine, cooked bulgur, or kasha.

Makes 6 servings

**Calories: 122   Protein: 4 g   Total fat: 5 g   Saturated fat: trace
Sodium: 611 mg**

Source: *Jenny Matthau, N.Y.*

TOFU SOUTH OF THE BORDER ENCHILADAS

½ cup chopped onions

¾ cup chopped sweet green pepper

4 ounces mild green chilies, fresh or canned, seeded, chopped, and drained

1 garlic clove, minced

½ teaspoon ground cumin seed

1 teaspoon dried cilantro

12 ounces firm tofu, drained and mashed

2 cups diced fresh tomatoes, drained and seeded

8 (8-inch) whole wheat tortillas

2 cups thick tomato salsa

½ cup shredded low-fat Cheddar cheese

1. Preheat the oven to 350°F.
2. In a bowl, combine the onions, peppers, chilies, garlic, cumin, cilantro, tofu, and diced tomatoes. Place ½ cup of the mixture in the center of each tortilla and roll up.
3. Place in an oiled baking dish, seam side down. Pour the salsa over the enchiladas. Sprinkle with shredded cheese.

Cover the pan with aluminum foil and bake for 25 to 30 minutes.

Serves 8

Calories: 189   Total fat: 7 g   Cholesterol: 4 mg   Sodium: 409 mg

Source: *Minnesota Soybean Research & Promotion Council*

VERY SPECIAL TEMPEH STEW

1 leek, whites and 2 inches of green, cut in half lengthwise, cleaned, and thinly sliced crosswise

6 garlic cloves, minced

¼ cup extra-virgin olive oil

2 carrots, peeled and cut in half-moons

2 potatoes, peeled and diced

2 celery stalks, thickly sliced

½ teaspoon sea salt or vegetable salt

1 large red or yellow tomato, seeds squeezed out, chopped

1 small red onion, chopped

½ red pepper, diced small

1 cup loosely packed chopped fresh cilantro

½ pound tempeh, any variety, cut in ¾-inch cubes

2 tablespoons barley miso dissolved in 1 cup hot water

⅓ cup dry white wine, sake, or sherry

1. In a heavy 4-quart pot, sauté the leek and 4 minced garlic cloves in 2 tablespoons of the oil for about 1 minute. Add the carrots, potatoes, celery, and sea salt and continue to sauté for 3 minutes longer. Cover the pot, lower the flame to minimum, and allow the vegetables to "sweat," or release their liquid.

2. Add the tomato, red onion, red pepper, and cilantro to the pot and stir. Replace the cover.

3. In a skillet, heat the remaining 2 tablespoons of oil. Add the remaining garlic, stir a few times, then add the tempeh and brown lightly on all sides, about 5 to 8 minutes.

4. Add the dissolved miso to the skillet and simmer until almost all the liquid has evaporated. Transfer the tempeh to the vegetable pot and, still on heat, deglaze the skillet with the wine, stirring to remove the browned bits, then add this to the vegetable pot as well.

5. Stir and continue to cook for a few more minutes. Serve hot atop rice, noodles, or a grain of your choice.

Makes 6 servings

Calories: 230   Protein: 11 g   Total fat: 12 g   Saturated fat: 2 g
Sodium: 419 mg

Source: *Roberta Atti Robinson, N.J.*

Side Dishes / Breakfast

SCRAMBLED CURRIED TOFU

1 small onion, minced
½ red pepper, diced small
2 tablespoons sesame oil
½ teaspoon turmeric
½ teaspoon ground cumin

¼ teaspoon curry powder, or more to taste
1 pound soft tofu
½ teaspoon sea salt, or to taste

1. In a large skillet, sauté the onion and red pepper in the sesame oil until the onion is translucent, about 2 to 3 minutes. Add the turmeric, cumin, and curry, stir well, and sauté 1 minute more.

2. With the skillet still on the heat, add the tofu and break up with a wooden spoon until crumbled throughout. Stir continuously over medium heat for another 5 to 6 minutes, making sure all the ingredients are thoroughly mixed to resemble scrambled eggs. Season with salt and serve immediately with whole grain toast for a high-protein, cholesterol-free breakfast.

Makes 4 servings

Calories: 157   Protein: 9 g   Total fat: 12 g   Saturated fat: 2 g
Sodium: 276 mg

TEMPEH SAUSAGE

Serve as an entrée with rice and steamed vegetables or in pita bread sandwiches with lettuce, tomato, and sprouts.

8-ounce package tempeh, cut crosswise into 4 rectangles

1 garlic clove, minced

2 tablespoons water

1 tablespoon canola oil

2 tablespoons natural soy sauce (shoyu or tamari)

2 tablespoons oat flour

½ teaspoon ground sage

¼ teaspoon dried marjoram

¼ teaspoon dried thyme

¼ teaspoon paprika

Pinch of cayenne

½ teaspoon fennel seeds

A few grinds of black pepper

½ cup cornmeal for dredging

2 tablespoons oil for frying

1. Steam the tempeh in a steamer for 20 minutes. Cool. Grate finely into a large bowl.
2. Add the garlic, water, canola oil, soy sauce, oat flour, and all the herbs and spices to the tempeh. Mix well. Make

walnut-size balls and press into patties; place these on a separate plate.

3. Place the cornmeal in a soup or pie plate. Dredge each patty in the cornmeal and place on a clean plate.

4. Fry the patties in oil on each side until well browned.

Makes 12 patties

Calories: 151   Protein: 9 g   Total fat: 9 g   Saturated fat: trace
Sodium: 350 mg

Source: *Jenny Matthau, N.Y.*

GRILLED TEMPEH

Serve with minestrone and a green salad for a light lunch or in sandwiches with lettuce and tomato.

1 package Seasoned Tempeh   *1 teaspoon canola oil*
(page 137), cut in half hori-
zontally, then across into 4
pieces (for a total of 8)

1. Heat an indoor or outdoor grill.

2. Brush the tempeh with the oil and grill on both sides until heated through, about 3 to 4 minutes per side.

Makes 2 to 4 servings

Calories: 104   Protein: 12 g   Total fat: 5 g   Saturated fat: .5 g
Sodium: 264 mg

SPINACH IN CREAMY WHITE SAUCE

2 tablespoons safflower or soy oil

2 tablespoons unbleached white flour

1 cup plain soy milk

½ teaspoon sea salt

2 garlic cloves, pressed

2 teaspoons mirin (sweet rice wine) or sherry

1/16 teaspoon grated fresh nutmeg

1 pound fresh spinach, washed

1. In a heavy saucepan, heat the oil and add the flour, stirring constantly for 3 to 5 minutes, or until the flour bubbles and becomes aromatic. Whisk in the soy milk, then stir constantly as the sauce thickens.

2. Add the salt, garlic, and rice wine or sherry. Simmer over low heat, uncovered, stirring occasionally, for 5 to 10 minutes. Remove from the heat and stir in the nutmeg, making sure it's well blended.

3. Place the wet spinach in a small pot, covered, and steam for 5 minutes, or until wilted. Drain and chop finely; add to the cream sauce and blend. Serve hot as a side dish or over rice or pasta.

Makes 6 servings (about 1½ cups)

Calories: 82   Protein: 4 g   Total fat: 6 g   Saturated fat: trace
Sodium: 242 mg

MOCK EGG SALAD

Serve in whole wheat pita bread with sprouts and tomato wedges.

12 ounces firm tofu, drained

2 teaspoons apple cider vinegar

1 teaspoon maple syrup or honey

2 teaspoons prepared mustard

1 teaspoon turmeric

1 teaspoon sea salt

1 tablespoon canola or olive oil

3 tablespoons finely diced celery

2 scallions, finely sliced

1 tablespoon finely chopped fresh parsley

¼ teaspoon freshly ground pepper, or to taste

1. Crumble the tofu into a medium bowl.

2. Combine the vinegar, maple syrup, mustard, turmeric, salt, and oil in a small bowl, then add to the tofu, stirring with a fork and breaking up lumps.

3. Add the celery, scallions, parsley, and pepper, stirring well. Chill in the refrigerator for 1 hour or more.

Makes about 4 servings

Calories: 107   Protein: 7 g   Total fat: 8 g   Saturated fat: trace
Sodium: 578 mg

CARROTS IN MISO SAUCE

1 tablespoon extra-virgin olive oil

1 small onion, minced

1 pound thin carrots, cut on the diagonal in ½-inch slices (about 2½ or 3 cups)

2 tablespoons mellow yellow miso

¾ cup vegetable stock or water

1 teaspoon lemon zest or 2 teaspoons orange zest (preferably organically grown)

1 teaspoon grated fresh gingerroot

Freshly ground black pepper to taste

1. In a medium saucepan, heat the oil, add the onion and carrots, and sauté over low heat for about 7 to 8 minutes, stirring often, until the carrot's earthy aroma mellows.

2. In a small bowl, combine the miso, stock, lemon or or-

ange zest, and gingerroot. Add to the carrots, cover, and simmer for 10 minutes. Remove the cover and cook another 10 minutes, until much of the liquid evaporates and the carrots are covered with a thickish miso sauce. Season with pepper and serve hot.

Makes 5 to 6 servings

Calories: 66   Protein: 1 g   Total fat: 3 g   Saturated fat: trace
Sodium: 177 mg

HIZIKI WITH MUSHROOMS AND TOFU

4 large dried shiitake mushrooms

3 cups warm water

½ cup dry hiziki seaweed

1 teaspoon sesame oil

8 ounces firm tofu, cubed

2 tablespoons natural soy sauce (shoyu or tamari), or to taste

Freshly ground pepper

1. Soak the mushrooms in 1½ cups water for 10 minutes, then remove the stems and chop. Soak the hiziki in the rest of the water for 10 minutes. Reserve the mushroom soaking liquid.
2. In a large skillet, sauté the hiziki in the oil, then add the mushrooms and the mushroom soaking liquid. Simmer for 15 minutes, covered.
3. Add the tofu and soy sauce, stir, and simmer another 15 minutes. Serve hot, with a grinding or two of pepper.

Makes 4 servings

Calories: 30   Protein: 1 g   Total fat: 1 g   Saturated fat: trace
Sodium: 524 mg

Sauces / Dips

HENRY'S MUSHROOM SAUCE

1 large onion, chopped

4 garlic cloves, minced

2 tablespoons extra-virgin olive oil

2 teaspoons dried thyme

1 teaspoon sea salt

½ teaspoon white pepper

2 pounds white mushrooms, cleaned and sliced

½ cup unbleached white flour

4 tablespoons white miso dissolved in 3 cups hot water

½ cup white wine (optional)

3 tablespoons kuzu or arrowroot powder dissolved in ½ cup cold water

1 to 2 tablespoons natural soy sauce (shoyu or tamari), or to taste

Chopped fresh parsley for garnish

1. In a heavy 4-quart pot, sauté the onions and garlic in the oil for 1 minute, then add the thyme, sea salt, and pepper. Continue to sauté until the onions are translucent, then add the mushrooms, stir, cover, lower the heat, and cook for about 10 minutes.

2. Sprinkle the flour over the mixture, making sure the onions and mushrooms are evenly coated. Add the miso water and wine if using and stir. Cover and simmer 5 minutes longer.

3. Stir the dissolved kuzu or arrowroot and add to the mushroom mixture. Stir continuously until the liquid thickens. Add a little more water if it is too thick or add more kuzu or arrowroot (always dissolved in a little cold

water first) if it is too thin. Add the soy sauce, garnish with parsley, and serve on top of millet, rice, quinoa, or Seasoned Tempeh.

Makes about 6 cups

Calories: 87   Protein: 3 g   Total fat: 3 g   Saturated fat: trace
Sodium: 528 mg

Source: *Roberta Atti Robinson, N.J.*

MISO PESTO SAUCE

4 cups loosely packed fresh basil leaves

¼ cup extra-virgin olive oil

1 or 2 garlic cloves, pushed through a garlic press

2 tablespoons barley miso

½ cup fresh shelled walnuts (make sure they smell fresh, not rancid)

1. Place the basil, oil, garlic, and barley miso in a food processor or blender and process until smooth.
2. Place the walnuts in a paper or plastic bag and beat a few times with a can or rolling pin to break them up. Add to the blender or processor and process 15 to 30 seconds, just to mix.

Makes about ¾ to 1 cup. Serve 1 or 2 tablespoons per bowl of freshly cooked hot pasta.

Calories: 128   Protein: 2 g   Total fat: 12 g   Saturated fat:1 g
Sodium: 170 mg

TOFU-GINGER DRESSING

½ teaspoon finely grated fresh gingerroot

8 ounces soft or silken tofu

1 teaspoon sea salt

¼ cup water

2 tablespoons olive oil

2 tablespoons balsamic or apple cider vinegar

Combine all the ingredients in a blender and puree until creamy. Serve over romaine lettuce or other salad greens.

Makes about 1¼ cups

Calories: 50   Protein: 2 g   Total fat: 5 g   Saturated fat: trace
Sodium: 269 mg

CILANTRO SAUCE

Serve over burritos or rice, or as a dip for vegetables.

3 tablespoons extra-virgin olive oil

2 cups finely chopped onions (about 3 onions)

Pinch of sea salt

3 tablespoons mashed garlic

2 cups cilantro leaves, tough stalks removed, washed and chopped

½ cup fresh parsley leaves, finely chopped

2 teaspoons dried basil

2½ tablespoons white or yellow miso (or to taste) diluted in 1 cup water

1 tablespoon lemon juice

1 tablespoon rice wine vinegar

1. In a large skillet or 2-quart saucepan, heat the olive oil over medium heat and sauté the onions with the salt until sweet and translucent, about 5 to 7 minutes. Add the garlic and sauté a few minutes more.

2. Add the chopped cilantro, parsley, and basil to the pot and mix well. Add the diluted miso, stir, and cook for

about 2 minutes more. Add the lemon juice and vinegar. Process briefly in the blender or food processor, in batches if needed.

Makes about 2 cups

Calories: 40   Protein: trace   Total fat: 3 g   Saturated fat: trace
Sodium: 117 mg

Source: *Melanie Ferreira, N.Y.*

TOFU-DILL SOUR CREAM

This is good in borscht or carrot soup, over steamed vegetables, or as a dip for raw vegetables.

6 ounces tofu, blanched and cooled

2 tablespoons lemon juice

1 teaspoon sea salt

1 tablespoon canola oil

¼ cup water

2 to 3 tablespoons chopped fresh dill

Place all the ingredients in a blender or food processor and blend until smooth. Alternatively, reserve the dill, blend the rest of the ingredients, and then stir in the dill for a flecked look.

Makes about 1 cup

Calories: 31   Protein: 2 g   Total fat: 3 g   Saturated fat: trace
Sodium: 269 mg

Source: *Melanie Ferreira, N.Y.*

Desserts

ALWAYS READY SOY AND WHEAT BRAN MUFFINS

1 cup boiling water

3 cups unprocessed wheat bran

2 tablespoons vinegar or lemon juice

2 cups low-fat vanilla-flavored soy milk

1 cup brown sugar

2 eggs, beaten

6 tablespoons soy oil

1½ cups unbleached white flour

1 cup defatted soy flour, sifted

2½ teaspoons baking soda

1 teaspoon salt

1. Preheat the oven to 400°F.

2. In a large bowl, pour the boiling water over 1 cup wheat bran; set aside for 5 minutes. In a small bowl, stir the vinegar or lemon juice into the soy milk and set aside for 5 minutes. The soy milk will begin to curdle.

3. Add the soy milk, brown sugar, beaten eggs, and soy oil to the soaked wheat bran and mix well. Add the remaining wheat bran, white flour, soy flour, baking soda, and salt to the mixture. Mix well. Spoon into oiled or sprayed muffin cups, filling two-thirds full. Bake for 20 to 22 minutes or until a toothpick inserted in the middle comes out clean.

Makes 24 muffins or 48 mini muffins

(per muffin)
Calories: 130   Protein: 5 g   Total fat: 5 g   Sodium: 120 mg
Cholesterol: 18 mg

Source: *The Soyfoods Council of America*

CRANAPPLE SNACK BARS

1 cup honey

3 tablespoons orange juice

1 teaspoon salt

⅓ cup soy oil

1 (10.5-ounce) package
silken tofu

1 teaspoon vanilla extract

1 egg

2 cups unbleached white flour

1 teaspoon baking soda

1 teaspoon cinnamon

2 cups peeled apple slices

2½ cups fresh or frozen
cranberries

½ cup chopped walnuts

1. Preheat the oven to 350 °F. Oil or spray a 10 × 15 × 1-inch baking pan.
2. In a large bowl, whip the honey, orange juice, and salt together, then blend in the oil. Add the tofu, vanilla, and egg and beat well.
3. In a separate bowl, sift together the flour, baking soda, and cinnamon. Add to the honey/oil mixture and stir well.
4. Fold in the apples, cranberries, and nuts. Pour the batter into the prepared pan and bake for 30 to 35 minutes, or until a toothpick inserted near the center comes out clean.

Makes 24 to 36 bars

Calories: 72   Protein: 1 g   Total fat: 3 g   Saturated fat: 0.4 g
Sodium: 88 mg   Cholesterol: 5 mg

Source: *Ohio Soybean Council*

GINGER PEACHY TOFRUITY

2 tablespoons agar flakes

½ cup water

⅓ cup maple crystals or natural
brown sugar

1 (1-pound 3-ounce) package silken tofu

2 tablespoons ginger juice (see Note) or ¼ cup chopped crystallized ginger

⅛ teaspoon sea salt

1 (20-ounce) package individually quick-frozen sliced peaches (about 4 cups)

Thin shreds ("needles") of fresh or crystallized ginger for garnish (optional)

1. In a small saucepan, place the agar and water and let sit for 5 minutes. Bring to a boil, then simmer until the agar is completely dissolved, about 5 minutes. Stir in the maple crystals or brown sugar until dissolved. Remove from the heat.

2. Place half the tofu, the ginger juice, sea salt, and fruit in a blender cup. When the agar mixture is ready, start the blender and pour in half the agar mixture in a thin stream. Blend until the mixture is smooth and without lumps, about 2 to 3 minutes. The mixture will look like soft frozen yogurt. Transfer to a bowl and place the bowl in the freezer. Repeat with the other half of the ingredients and add to the bowl. Serve immediately or keep in the freezer for up to 20 minutes, loosely covered. Do not freeze.

3. Scoop into 6 dessert cups, garnish with ginger shreds if using, and serve.

Makes 6 servings

**Calories: 142   Protein: 7 g   Total fat: 4 g   Saturated fat: trace
Sodium: 297 mg**

Note: To make ginger juice, grate 2 to 3 inches of ginger—no need to peel—and squeeze the gratings by hand, in cheesecloth, or in a garlic press to obtain the ginger juice.

Source: *Jeri DeLoach Jackson, N.Y.*

JALAPEÑO BLUE CORN BREAD OR MUFFINS

2½ teaspoons aluminum-free baking powder

¼ teaspoon sea salt

2 cups blue cornmeal or freshly ground yellow cornmeal

1½ cups corn kernels, preferably fresh

1 egg, preferably organic

3 tablespoons melted butter or cold-pressed safflower oil

1 cup plain soy milk

1 tablespoon maple syrup

1 fresh jalapeño pepper, seeded and finely chopped

1. Preheat the oven to 425 °F. Oil or butter a 9×9-inch baking pan or muffin pan.
2. In a large bowl, mix together the baking powder, sea salt, and cornmeal. Blend thoroughly. Add the corn kernels.
3. In another bowl, beat the egg until fluffy, then whisk in the butter or oil, the soy milk, the maple syrup, and the jalapeño pepper.
4. Pour the liquid ingredients into the cornmeal mixture and combine quickly; do not overbeat or the corn bread will be dry. Pour into the prepared pan and bake for 20 to 25 minutes, or until a knife inserted comes out clean.

Makes 1 loaf or 12 muffins

Calories: 136   Protein: 3 g   Total fat: 5 g   Saturated fat: 2 g
Cholesterol: 25 mg   Sodium: 133 mg

ORANGE SHERBET

1½ cups fresh orange juice with pulp

1 tablespoon grated orange rind

1½ cups plain or vanilla soy milk

¼ cup frozen orange juice concentrate

1. Combine all the ingredients in a large bowl or pitcher. Chill for at least 1 hour.
2. Freeze the mixture in an ice cream maker according to the manufacturer's directions about 1 hour before serving.

Makes about 1 quart (8 servings)

**Calories: 50   Protein: 2 g   Total fat: 1 g   Saturated fat: trace
Sodium: 6 mg**

Source: *The Soyfoods Association of America*

PORTUGUESE RICE PUDDING

1½ cups plain soy milk
½ teaspoon sea salt
4 to 6 tablespoons maple syrup
1 tablespoon canola oil
1 teaspoon vanilla extract

½ teaspoon grated lemon rind
2 cups cooked brown or white rice
⅓ cup raisins (optional)
Ground cinnamon

1. In a bowl, mix the soy milk, salt, maple syrup, oil, vanilla, and lemon rind; whisk until well combined. Add the rice and raisins if using.
2. Transfer the rice mixture to a heavy pot, bring to a boil, and simmer, covered, for approximately 20 minutes, stirring occasionally. Remove from the heat and place in individual serving dishes, garnishing with a shake or two of cinnamon. Serve hot or cold.

Makes 6 servings

**Calories: 184   Protein: 3.5 g   Total fat: 4 g   Saturated fat: 0.3 g
Sodium: 191 mg**

Source: *Melanie Ferreira, N.Y.*

SWEET CHERRY FREEZE DESSERT

3 cups fresh or frozen sweet cherries (Bing cherries)

¼ cup frozen apple juice concentrate

1 cup low-fat vanilla soy milk

Puree all the ingredients in a blender or food processor until well blended. Freeze in an ice cream maker according to the manufacturer's instructions about 1 hour before serving.

Makes about 1 quart (8 servings)

Calories: 63   Protein: 1.5 g   Total fat: 1 g   Saturated fat: trace Sodium: 6 mg

Source: *The Soyfoods Association of America*

TOFU CREAM PIE

1 prepared piecrust

2 pounds soft tofu

3 tablespoons tahini (sesame paste)

Grated rind of 1 lemon (preferably organically grown)

1 tablespoon lemon juice

½ cup maple syrup

2 teaspoons vanilla extract

1. Prebake the crust in a 350°F. oven for 5 minutes.
2. Crumble the tofu into a blender or food processor. Add the tahini, lemon rind, juice, maple syrup, and vanilla and process until smooth and creamy, stopping the machine several times to scrape the mixture down the sides.
3. Pour the tofu mixture into the center of the prebaked crust, allowing the filling to radiate outward. Shake gently

to distribute, but do not use any spreader. Bake at 350°F.
for 35 to 40 minutes. Allow to cool before slicing.

Makes 1 pie (12 servings)

Calories: 185   Protein: 7 g   Total fat: 10 g   Saturated fat: 2 g
Sodium: 100 mg

Glossary

Amino acids. Building blocks of proteins and neurotransmitters. There are about twenty amino acids, eight of which are called essential because the body cannot synthesize them so they must be obtained from food. Combinations of B_6 are used to treat splitting, peeling nails. Arginine, lysine, and phenylalanine were banned by the FDA from over-the-counter diet pills on February 10, 1992.

Antagonist. A drug, hormone, or neurotransmitter that blocks a response from a receptor site.

Antioxidant. Prevents oxidation—the combining with oxygen—of substances. Rancidity of fats and rust are examples of oxidation. Antioxidants include vitamins C and E and zinc.

Atherosclerosis. A form of arteriosclerosis. The inner layers of the artery walls are made thick and irregular by deposits of a fatty substance. The internal channel of the arteries becomes narrowed, reducing the blood supply.

Bioflavonoids. Sometimes called vitamin P. Coloring compounds such as rutin, esculin, and tangeretin in plants. Bioflavonoids have various biological activities in mammals and are being studied to determine if they have anticancer and blood vessel protection properties.

Biotechnology. The use of living cells or parts of cells to perform procedures and to make products.

Bowman-Birk Inhibitor (BBI). A nonnutritive substance in soy that is a protease inhibitor (see) and helps block the growth of certain cancers.

Calcium. The adult body contains about three pounds of calcium, 99 percent of which provides hardness for bones and teeth. Approximately 1 percent of calcium is distributed in body fluids where it is essential for normal cell activity. If the body does not get enough calcium from food, it steals the mineral from bones. Abnormal loss of calcium from bones weakens them and makes them porous or brittle and susceptible to fractures. Calcium deficiencies can result in osteopenia (less bone than normal, a condition preceding osteoporosis) and osteoporosis (a severe decrease in bone mass with diagnosable fractures), which affects 25 percent of women after menopause. The percentage of calcium absorption declines progressively with age. The RDA for calcium is 1000 milligrams for adults. There is also some evidence that an intake of about 1000 milligrams of calcium may protect against hypertension or high blood pressure.

Carbohydrate. Starches and sugars contain a high proportion of carbohydrates. These are chemicals that contain carbon, hydrogen, and oxygen. Gums and mucilages are complex carbohydrates and are often ingredients in soothing herbs and medications.

Carcinogen. A substance that causes cancer.

Carcinogenesis. The development of cancer.

Carcinoma. A malignant tumor that grows from epithelial tissue (see Epithelium).

Cardiovascular. Pertaining to the heart and blood vessels.

Cholesterol. A fat-soluble, crystalline steroid alcohol occurring in animal fats and oils, nervous tissue, egg yolk, and blood. It is important in metabolism but has been implicated as contributing to hardening and clogging of the arteries and subsequently heart attacks.

Coronary artery disease. The arteries that carry blood become narrowed.

Coronary thrombosis. A blood clot in one of the arteries that carries blood from the heart. Often called a "heart attack."

Daidzein. A soybean estrogen (isoflavone) that appears to have cancer-fighting potential.

Daily values. The U.S. government has changed the standards for the intake of vitamins, minerals, and other nutrients. Since May 1994, the labeling on foods has been changed to Daily Values.

Daily Values (DV) comprise two sets of references for nutrients, Daily Reference Values (DRVs) and Reference Daily Intakes (RDIs).

Daily Reference Values (DRVs) are for nutrients for which no set of standards previously existed, such as fat, cholesterol, carbohydrate, protein, and fiber. DRVs for these energy-producing nutrients are based on the number of calories consumed per day. For labeling purposes, 2000 calories has been established as the reference for calculating percent Daily Values. This level was chosen in part because many health experts say it approximates the maintenance calorie requirements of the group most often targeted for weight reduction: postmenopausal women.

DRVs for the energy-producing nutrients are calculated as follows:

- Fat based on 30 percent of calories.
- Saturated fat based on 10 percent of calories.
- Carbohydrate based on 60 percent of calories.
- Protein based on 10 percent of calories.
- Fiber based on 11.5 grams of fiber per 1000 calories.

The DRVs for cholesterol, sodium, and potassium, which do not contribute calories, remain the same no matter what the calorie level.

Reference Daily Intakes (RDIs) are a set of dietary references based on and replacing the Recommended Dietary Allowances (RDAs) for essential vitamins and minerals and, in selected groups, protein. You will continue to see vitamins and minerals expressed as percentages on the label but these figures now refer to the Daily Values.

DNA (deoxyribonucleic acid). The complex substance that makes up genes; it contains the genetic information for all organisms.

Enzymes. Substances in the body necessary for accomplishing chemical changes such as processing sugar to create energy or breaking down food in the intestines for digestion.

Epidemiological study. A study that measures the incidence of disease in large population groups and looks for associations with various genetic or environmental factors.

Epithelium. The cellular covering of internal and external body surfaces, including the lining of vessels and small cavities. The epithelium consists of cells joined by small amounts of cementing substances and is classified according to the number of layers and shape of the cells.

Equol. A soy estrogen identified in 1982 similar to the human estrogen, estradiol-17. It has been found to be elevated in the urine of people who eat soy foods.

Estrogen. A hormone produced by the ovaries that is mainly responsible for female sexual characteristics. Estrogen influences bone mass by slowing or halting bone loss, improving the retention of calcium by the kidney, and improving the absorption of dietary calcium by the intestine. Estrogen is given to relieve menopausal symptoms, prevent or relieve aging changes in the vagina and urethra, and to help prevent osteoporosis (see).

Fatty acids. Compounds of carbon, hydrogen, and oxygen that combine with glycerol to make fats.

Fiber. Found in whole grains and many vegetables, fiber helps speed cancer-causing compounds through the digestive system. It discourages the growth of harmful bacteria while bolstering healthful ones, and it may encourage production of a healthier form of estrogen.

Flavonoids. Compounds in plants such as pigments. Most plants and vegetables contain flavonoids. Bioflavonoids have biological effects. Rutin, for example, has chelating properties and influences the functioning of minute blood vessels. It is believed that flavonoids block receptor sites for certain hormones that promote cancers.

Free radicals. Highly reactive molecules generated when a cell "burns" its foods with oxygen to fuel life processes. Free radicals act like "loose cannons" rolling around and damaging cells. This damage is thought to be a first step in cancer development. Antioxidants such as vitamins C and E and a number of phytochemicals found in food can suppress free radical cell damage.

g or **gm.** Abbreviation for gram, a small metric measure equal to 1/1000 kilograms or 0.03527 ounce.

Gene. The smallest genetic unit of a chromosome. It is a piece of DNA that contains the hereditary information for the production of a protein.

Genetic engineering. The technique of removing, modifying, or adding genetic material in living cells to produce a new substance or new function. This includes adding or deleting genes as well as preventing or turning off the expression of particular genes.

Genistein. A plant estrogen found in the urine of people with diets rich in soybeans and, to a lesser extent, in the cabbage family vegetables. This compound seems to block the growth of new blood vessels, which is essential for some tumors to grow and spread.

Glucose. Sugar that occurs naturally in blood, grapes, and corn. A source of energy for animals and plants. Sweeter then sucrose, it is used medicinally for nutritional purposes and in the treatment of diabetic coma. It is also used topically to soothe the skin.

Glucosides. Sugar compounds usually containing an alcohol.

Glycosides. A class of drugs used in heart failure. Many flowering plants contain cardiac glycosides. The most well known are foxglove, lily of the valley, and squill. The cardiac glycosides have the ability to increase the force and power of the heartbeat without increasing the amount of oxygen needed by the heart muscle. Among the glycosides are cyanogens, goitrogens, estrogens, and saponins. They are found in soybeans as well as most legumes.

HDL. Abbreviation for high-density lipoprotein (see).

High-Density Lipoprotein (HDL). The "good" cholesterol that is believed to pick up excess cholesterol in the blood and help the body eliminate it.

Hypoglycemia. Low blood sugar—the opposite of diabetes.

Initiation. An event that alters the genetic code of a cell or causes some other basic, permanent damage, predisposing that cell to become a cancer cell later. Chemical carcinogens, viruses, radiation, and other factors are thought to be capable of causing initiation.

Isoflavones. Natural plant estrogens found in soy.

ISP. Abbreviation for isolated soy protein (see page 100).

LDL. Abbreviation for low-density lipoprotein (see).

Legumes. Plants that include seeds in a pod, such as beans and peas. The *Leguminosae* family includes over 18,000 species and is one of the most economically important plant families in the world. They include the phytochemicals being studied as nutraceuticals. Phytochemicals from legumes are already utilized as food additives, fungicides, and anticancer agents.

Lignin. Binding agent in animal feed from plant fibers. There is no reported use of the chemical and no toxicology information available.

Linoleic acid. An essential fatty acid (see) prepared from edible fats and oils. Component of vitamin F and a major constituent of many vegetable oils, for example, cottonseed and soybean. Used in emulsifiers and vitamins. Large doses can cause nausea and vomiting.

Linolenic acid. Polyunsaturated acid produced in the body as a metabolite of linoleic acid. A nutrient used in the treatment of eczema. Alpha-linolenic acid in the diet of Mediterranean people is believed to be important in the prevention of heart disease.

Low-Density Lipoprotein (LDL). The "bad" cholesterol that is believed to collect cholesterol in the blood and deposit it in the cells.

Lysine. An essential amino acid found in soy but usually missing in other food plants.

MAO Inhibitors. *See* Monoamine oxidase inhibitors.

Metastasis. Transfer of disease from one organ or part of the body to another not directly connected with it.

mg. Abbreviation for milligram, which is one-thousandth of a gram.

mg/dl. Milligrams per deciliter of blood.

Minerals. Inorganic materials found in the earth's crust.

Monoamine oxidase. An enzyme that acts in the nervous system to break down certain types of neurotransmitters (chemical messengers sent between nerve cells) such as dopamine, norepinephrine, and serotonin.

Monoamine Oxidase Inhibitors (MAOIs). A class of antidepressant medications usually prescribed for people who have not responded to tricyclics or who have certain forms of depression with symptoms including an increase in weight, appetite, or sleep. MAOIs may also be used for cases of mixed anxiety and depression, depression accompanied by pain, panic disorder, posttraumatic stress disorder, and bipolar depression. The drugs raise the level of neurotransmitters by preventing their destruction by enzymes. People taking MAOIs must adhere to a special diet because of the interaction of the medications with certain foods. Foods that contain tyramine such as cheeses, yogurt, sour cream, beef or chicken livers, and red wines should be avoided. The combination of MAOIs and tyramine can shoot up blood pressure to dangerous levels. Symptoms include headache, increased or decreased heart rate, nausea and vomiting, sweating, fever or cold clammy skin, and chest pain.

Neurotransmitters. Molecules that carry chemical messages between nerve cells. Neurotransmitters are released from a nerve cell, diffuse across the minute distance between two nerve cells (synaptic cleft), and bind to a receptor at another nerve site.

Osteoporosis. A condition characterized by low bone mass and an increased susceptibility to bone fractures.

Phenolic acids (tannins). Found in parsley, carrots, broccoli, cabbage, tomatoes, eggplant, peppers, citrus fruits, whole grains, and berries, they have antioxidant properties, inhibit formation of nitrosamine, a cancer-causing agent, and affect enzyme activity.

Phytic acid. Occurs in nature in the seeds of soy and cereal grains and is derived commercially from corn. It is used to chelate heavy metals, as a rust inhibitor, in metal cleaning, and in the treatment of hard water.

Phytoestrogens. A host of estrogens, including genistein and daidzein, which have been identified in plants. Although they are considerably less active than those in animals, they have been reported to protect against a number of cancers including prostate, breast, colon, melanoma, and others. Chronic exposure may lead to the accumulation of levels that are active in humans. *See also* Genistein.

Plant estrogens. *See* Phytoestrogens.

Plant sterols. Vitamin D precursors found in broccoli, cabbage, cucumbers, squash, yams, tomatoes, eggplant, peppers, soy products, and whole grains that cause cells to differentiate.

Plasma. The fluid portion of the blood or lymph that carries in solution a wide range of ions, minerals, vitamins, antibodies, proteins, enzymes, and/or other essential substances.

Precursor. A biologic process in which a substance turns into another active or more mature substance. Beta-carotene is a precursor of vitamin A because the body can use it to make vitamin A.

Promotion. An intermediate stage of cancer development during which initiated (see) cells, in the presence of promoters, move further along the pathway to cancer. The promotion stage may take several decades in humans.

Prostaglandins (PGA, PGB, PGC, PGD). A group of extremely potent hormonelike substances present in many tissues. There are more than sixteen known with effects such as dilating or constricting blood vessels, stimulation of intestinal or bronchial smooth muscle, uterine stimulation, and antagonism to hormones and influencing fat metabolism. Various prostaglandins in the body can cause fever, inflammation, and headaches. Prostaglandins or drugs that affect prostaglandins are used medically to induce labor, prevent and treat peptic ulcers, control high blood pressure, treat bronchial asthma, and induce delayed menstruation.

Protease inhibitors. Compounds in soy and some other plants that inhibit enzymes involved in the growth of tumors.

Proteins. Organic compounds made up of amino acids. Proteins are one of the major constituents of plant and animal cells.

RDAs. *Recommended Dietary Allowances* of the Food and Nutrition Board, National Academy of Sciences, National Research Council. Has largely been replaced by *Daily Values* (see).

Receptor. A protein molecule that may also be composed of fat and carbohydrate that resides on the surface or in the nucleus of a cell and recognizes and binds a specific molecule of appropriate size, shape, and charge. Receptors are activated by specific nerve chemicals, hormones, or drugs and can be regarded as "biological locks" that can be "opened" only with specific keys.

Saponin. Any of numerous natural glycosides—natural or synthetic compounds derived from sugars—that occur in many plants such as soapbark, soapwort, or sarsaparilla. Characterized by their ability to foam in water, saponins are believed to reduce blood cholesterol. They can be beneficial or deleterious. They may be either steroidal or triterpenoid in structure.

Sterol. Any class of solid, complex alcohols from animals and plants. Cholesterol is a sterol.

Thrombus. A blood clot that forms within the heart or blood vessel and remains attached to its point of origin.

Thyroid. The thyroid is a butterfly-shaped gland located in the neck with a "wing" on either side of the windpipe. The gland produces thyroxine, which controls the rates of chemical reactions in the body. Generally, the more thyroxine, the faster the body works. Thyroxine needs iodine to function.

Tyramine. A derivative of tyrosine (see below), it is a chemical present in mistletoe and many common foods and beverages. It raises blood pressure but usually causes no problem because enzymes in the body hold it in check. When drugs are used that inhibit monoamine oxidase (MAO), the major enzyme that restrains its actions, blood pressure can shoot to dangerous levels if foods and beverages containing significant levels of tyramine are ingested. Some soybean products are among the foods that are high in tyramine.

Tyrosine. A widely distributed amino acid termed nonessential because it does not seem to be necessary for growth. A building block of protein, it is used as a dietary supplement.

Vitamins. Chemical compounds that are vital for growth, health, metabolism, and physical and mental well-being. Some vitamins aid enzymes—the workhorses of the body that perform chemical reactions. Other vitamins form parts of hormones—the directors sent out from glands to turn on other organs. There are two basic types of vitamins—fat-soluble and water-soluble. The fat-soluble vitamins such as A can accumulate in the body and cause problems if taken in excessive amounts. The water-soluble vitamins such as C cannot be stored to any great degree and must be obtained through foods.

Where to Get More Information

Beano. A product that helps stop gas some people may suffer from eating beans. Call 1-800-257-8650. In Canada call 1-800-668-8968 for information and a free sample.

Eden Foods Inc.
701 Tecumseh Rd.
Clinton, MI 49236
1-800-248-0320
FAX 1-517-456-6075

Write for a free issue of *Environmental Nutrition News Letter of Diet, Nutrition and Health* and subscription information.
Environmental Nutrition
PO Box 420451
Palm Coast, FL 32142-0451

Fearn Natural Foods
Modern Products
Milwaukee, WI 53209
Send a stamped self-addressed envelope for recipes using soy products.

Missouri Soybean Merchandising Council
PO Box 479
Columbus, OH 43216-0479
1-614-249-2492
Will provide recipe brochure.

The Natural Gourmet Institute for Food and Health
48 W. 21st St., 2nd floor
NY, NY 10010
1-212-645-5170
Cooking classes incorporate soybeans and other natural foods. Classes are held weekly for the general public. Career program requiring 600 hours is also available.

Natus, Inc.
2386 28th St.
Long Island City, NY 11105
For information about "Remedies of Natural Origin," genistein and daidzein, call 1-800-227-8454.

Soyfoods Association of America
One Sutter St., Suite 300
San Francisco, CA 94104
1-415-393-9697
FAX 1-415-433-9494

United Soybean Board
PO Box 419200
St. Louis, MO 63141-9200
A consumer help line for soy food information and recipes. Call 1-800-SOY-INFO (1-800-769-4636).

Vitasoy (USA) Inc.
99 Park La.
Brisbane, CA 94005
1-800-VITASOY (1-800-848-2769)
Offers recipes and information.

Worthington Foods, Inc.
900 Proprietors Rd.
Worthington, OH 43085
Will provide information on soy analogs and recipes.

References

Adams, Ruth. "Health Aspects of Soybean Products." *Better Nutrition for Today's Living* 55, 9 (September 1993): 44.

Adlercreutz, C. Herman. "Soybean Phytoestrogen Intake and Cancer Risk." Paper presented at The First International Symposium on the Role of Soy in Preventing and Treating Chronic Disease, Mesa, AZ, February 20–23, 1994.

Adlercreutz, C. H.; R. Heikkinen, and M. Woods et al. "Excretion of the Lignans Enterolactone and Enterodiol and of Equol in Omnivorous and Vegetarian Postmenopausal Women and in Women With Breast Cancer," *Lancet* (December 11, 1982): 1295–99.

Alberts, David, and Dava Garcia. "An Overview of Clinical Cancer Chemoprevention Studies with Emphasis on Positive Phase III Studies." Paper presented at The First International Symposium on the Role of Soy in Preventing and Treating Chronic Disease, Mesa, AZ, February 20–23, 1994.

American Heart Association. "Response to Media Coverage of Soy Protein Meta-Analysis Study." Dallas, TX, August 2, 1995.

Anderson, James, Bryan Johnstone, and Margaret Cook-Newell. "Meta-Analysis of the Effects of Soy Protein Intake on Serum Lipids." *New England Journal of Medicine* 333 (1995): 276–82.

Anderson, Robert, and Walter Wolf. "Compositional Changes in Trypsin Inhibitors, Phytic Acid, Saponins and Isoflavones Related to Soybean Processing." Paper presented at The First International

Symposium on the Role of Soy in Preventing and Treating Chronic Disease, Mesa, AZ, February 20–23, 1994.

Arnold, Kathryn. "The Joy of Soy." *The Natural Way* (August/September 1995): 58–59.

Ascherio, Alberto, and Walter Willett. "New Directions in Dietary Studies of Coronary Heart Disease." Paper presented at The First International Symposium on the Role of Soy in Preventing and Treating Chronic Disease, Mesa, Arizona, February 20–23, 1994.

Baird, Donna Day, et al. "Dietary Intervention Study to Assess Estrogenicity of Dietary Soy among Postmenopausal Women." *Journal of Clinical Endocrinology and Metabolism* 80 (1995): 1685–90.

Barnes, S., G. Peterson, C. Grubbs, and K. Setchell. "Potential Role of Dietary Isoflavones in the Prevention of Cancer." *Advances in Experimental Medicine and Biology* 354 (1994): 135–47.

Barnes, S., et al. "Soybeans Inhibit Mammary Tumors in Models of Breast Cancer." In *Mutagens and Carcinogens in the Diet*. New York: Wiley-Liss, 1990: 239–53.

Barnes, S. "Effect of Genistein on In Vitro and In Vivo Models of Cancer." Paper presented at The First International Symposium on the Role of Soy in Preventing and Treating Chronic Disease, Mesa, AZ, February 20–23, 1994.

Billings, P. C., P. M. Newberne, and A. R. Kennedy. "Protease Inhibitor Suppression of Colon and Anal Gland Carcinogenesis Induced by Dimethylhydrazine." *Carcinogenesis* 11, 7 (July 1990): 108–86.

Brennan, Jennifer. "The Emperor's Soy Sauce." *Gourmet* (January 1995): 92.

Bricklin, Mark, and the editors of *Prevention* Magazine. *Nutrition Advisor: The Complete, Up-to-Date Guide to Healthy Eating*. New York: MJF Books, 1993.

Brody, Jane. "Low-Fat Diet in Mice Slows Prostate Cancer." *New York Times* (October 18, 1995): C13.

Brown, K. H., F. Perez, J. Fadel, G. Brunsgaard, K. M. Ostrom, and W. C. MacLean Jr. "The Effect of Dietary Fiber (Soy Polysaccharide) on the Severity, Duration, and Nutritional Outcome of Acute, Watery Diarrhea in Children." *Pediatrics* 92, 2 (August 1993): 241–7.

Cassidy, A., S. Bingham, and K. D. R. Setchell. "Biological Effects of a Diet of Soy Protein Rich in Isoflavones on the Menstrual Cycle of

Premenopausal Women." *American Journal of Clinical Nutrition* 60, 3 (September 1994): 333–40.

Composition of Foods: Raw, Process, Prepared. 1989 Supplement. United States.

Coward, L., N. C. Barnes, K. D. R. Setchell, and S. Barnes. "Genistein, Daidzein and their B-glycoside Conjugates: Antitumor Isoflavones in Soybean Foods from American and Asian Diets." *Journal of Agricultural Food Chemistry* 41 (1993): 1961–67.

Cruz, M. L., et al. "Effects of Infant Nutrition on Cholesterol Synthesis Rates." *Pediatric Research* 35, 2 (February 1994): 135–40.

"Dietary Flavonoids and Risk of Coronary Heart Disease." Brief Critical Reviews. *Nutrition Reviews* 52, 2 (February 1994): 59–68.

Dwyer, Johanna. "Overview: Dietary Approaches for Reducing Cardiovascular Disease Risks." Paper presented at The First International Symposium on the Role of Soy in Preventing and Treating Chronic Disease, Mesa, AZ, February 20–23, 1994.

Dwyer, Johanna, Barry Goldin, Nora Saul, Lisa Gualtieri, Susan Barakat, and Herman Adlercreutz. "Tofu and Soy Drinks Contain Phytoestrogens." *Journal of the American Dietetic Association* 94, 7 (July 1994): 739.

Emmett, Jill, R. N., coordinator, University of Kentucky's Metabolic Research Group. Communication with author. 17–18 September 1995.

Erdman, John, Jr., and Elizabeth Fordyce. "Soy Products and the Human Diet." *American Journal of Clinical Nutrition* 49 (1989): 725–37.

Erdman, John, Jr. Personal communication with author. 7 September 1995.

Facchinetti, F. et al. "Oral Magnesium Successfully Relieves Premenstrual Mood Changes." *Obstetrics and Gynecology* 78 (1991): 177–81.

"First International Symposium on the Role of Soy in Preventing and Treating Chronic Disease." *The Journal of Nutrition* 125, 3S (March 1995): Supplement.

Ford, Barbara. *Future Food: Alternate Protein for the Year 2000.* New York: William Morrow, 1978.

Forsythe, William, III. "Soy Protein, Thyroid Regulation, and Cholesterol Metabolism." Paper presented at The First International Symposium on the Role of Soy in Preventing and Treating Chronic Disease, Mesa, AZ, February 20–23, 1994.

Fotsis, Theodore, et al. "Genistein, a Dietary Ingested Isoflavonoid, Inhibits Cell Proliferation and In Vitro Angiogenesis." Paper presented at The First International Symposium on the Role of Soy in Preventing and Treating Chronic Disease, Mesa, AZ, February 20–23, 1994.

Friedenwald, J., and J. Ruhrah. "The Use of the Soy Bean as a Food in Diabetes." *American Journal of Medical Science* 140 (1910): 793–803.

Gaby, Suzanne, Adrianne Bendich, Vishwa Singh, and Lawrence Machlin. *Vitamin Intake and Health: A Scientific Review.* New York: Marcel Dekker, Inc., 1991.

Golbitz, Peter. "Traditional Soyfoods: Processing and Products." Paper presented at The First International Symposium on the Role of Soy in Preventing and Treating Chronic Disease, Mesa, AZ, February 20–23, 1994.

Goldbeck, Nikki and David Goldbeck. *The Goldbecks' Guide to Good Foods.* New York: New American Library, 1987.

Goldberg, Anne Carol. "Perspectives on Soy Protein as a Nonpharmacological Approach for Lowering Cholesterol." Paper presented at The First International Symposium on the Role of Soy in Preventing and Treating Chronic Disease, Mesa, AZ, February 20–23, 1994.

Graf, E., and J. W. Eaton. "Suppression of Colonic Cancer by Dietary Phytic Acid." *Nutrition and Cancer* 19, 1 (1993): 11–9.

Hausman, Patricia, and Judith Hurley. *Healing Foods.* New York: Dell Publishing Co., 1991.

Hawrylewicz, E. J., Jose Zapata, and William Blair. "Soy and Experimental Cancer: Animal Studies." Paper presented at The First International Symposium on the Role of Soy in Preventing and Treating Chronic Disease, Mesa, AZ, February 20–23, 1994.

Hinds, G., N. P. Bell, D. McMaster, and D. R. McCluskey. "Normal Red Cell Magnesium Concentrations and Magnesium Loading Tests in Patients with Chronic Fatigue Syndrome." *Annals of Clinical Biochemistry* 31 (December 1994): 459–61.

Hodges, R. E., W. A. Krehl, D. B. Stone, and A. Lopez. "Dietary Carbohydrates and Low Cholesterol Diets: Effects on Serum Lipids of Man." *American Journal of Clinical Nutrition* 20 (1967): 198–208.

Howe, G., et al. "Dietary Intake of Fiber and Decreased Risk of Cancers of the Colon and Rectum: Evidence from Combined Analysis of 13 Case-Control Studies." *Journal of the National Cancer Institute* 84, 24 (December 16, 1992): 1887–96.

———. "Dietary Factors and the Risk of Breast Cancer." *Journal of the National Cancer Institute of Canada* 83, 20 (October 16, 1991): 1505–1507.

Hutchins, Andrea, Joanne Slavin, and Johanna Lampe. "Urinary Isoflavonoid Phytoestrogen and Lignan Excretion After Consumption of Fermented and Unfermented Soy Products." *Journal of American Dietetic Association* 95, 5 (May 1995): 545.

"Improving America's Diet and Health: From Recommendations to Action." A Report of the Committee on Dietary Guidelines Implementation. Food and Nutrition Board Institute of Medicine. Paul R. Thomas, editor. Washington, D.C.: National Academy Press, 1991.

Imura, T., T. Kanazawa, T. Watanabe, and Y. Fukushi, et al. "Hypotensive Effect of Soy Protein and Its Hydrolysate." *Annals of the New York Academy of Science* 676 (March 15, 1993): 327–30.

Jenkins, D. J. A. "A New Approach to the Dietary Management of Diabetes." *Diabetes Care* 5 (1982): 634–41.

Kanazawa, Takemichi, et al. "Protective Effects of Soy Protein on the Peroxidizability of Lipoproteins in Cerebrovascular Diseases." Paper presented at The First International Symposium on the Role of Soy in Preventing and Treating Chronic Disease, Mesa, AZ, February 20–23, 1994.

———, M. Tanaka, T. Uemura, T. Osanai, et al. "Anti-atherogenicity of Soybean Protein." *Annals of the New York Academy of Sciences* 676 (March 15, 1993): 202–14.

Kennedy, Ann. "The Evidence for Soybean Products as Cancer Preventive Agents." Paper presented at The First International Symposium on the Role of Soy in Preventing and Treating Chronic Disease, Mesa, AZ, February 20–23, 1994.

Kiguchi, K., et al. "Genistein-Induced Cell Differentiation and Protein-Linked DNA Strand Breakage in Human Melanoma Cells." *Cancer Communication* 2, 8 (1990): 271–77.

Kinoshita, E., et al. "Purification and Identification of an Angiotensin I-Converting Enzyme Inhibitor from Soy Sauce." *Bioscience Biotechnology and Biochemistry* 57, 7 (July 1993): 1107–10.

Klein, Barbara, A. K. Perry, and N. Adair. "Incorporating Soy Proteins into Baked Products for Use in Clinical Studies." *Journal of Nutrition* 125, 3 Suppl. (March 1995): 666S–74S.

Klein, Barbara. Personal communication with author. 6 September 1995.

Kritchevsky, David. "Dietary Protein, Cholesterol, and Atherosclerosis: A Review of the Early History." Paper presented at The First International Symposium on the Role of Soy in Preventing and Treating Chronic Disease, Mesa, AZ, February 20–23, 1994.

Lancaster, Teresa, clinical research assistant, University of Kentucky's Metabolic Research Group. Communication with author. 17 September 1995.

Liener, Irvin. "Possible Adverse Effects of Soybean Anticarcinogens." Paper presented at The First International Symposium on the Role of Soy in Preventing and Treating Chronic Disease, Mesa, AZ, February 20–23, 1994.

Lifshitz, Fima, ed. *Nutrition for Special Needs in Infancy: Protein Hydrolysates.* New York: Marcel Dekker, Inc., 1985.

Ling, W. H., and P. J. Jones. "Dietary Phytosterols: A Review of Metabolism, Benefits and Side Effects." *Life Science* 57, 3 (June 9, 1995): 195–206.

Lo, G. S. "Physiological Effects and Physico-chemical Properties of Soy Cotyledon Fiber." *Advances in Experimental Medicine and Biology* 270 (1990): 49–66.

Messina, M. J., V. Persky, K. D. Setchell, and S. Barnes. "Soy Intake and Cancer Risk: A Review of the In Vitro and In Vivo Data." *Nutrition and Cancer* 21, 2 (1994): 113–31.

Miettinen T. A., P. Puska, H. Gylling, H. Vanhanen, and E. Vartiainen. "Reduction of Serum Cholesterol with Sitostanol-ester Margarine in a Mildly Hypercholesterolemic Population." *New England Journal of Medicine* 333 (November 16, 1995): 1308–12.

Mirsalis, John. Personal communication with author. 13 September 1995.

Mortin, M. S., G. Wilcox, et al. "Determination of Lignans and Isoflavonoids in Human Female Plasma Following Dietary Supplementation." *Journal of Endocrinology* 142, 2 (August 1994): 251–59.

Nielsen, Forrest. "Boron—An Overlooked Element of Potential Nutritional Importance." *Nutrition Today* (January/February 1988): 4–7.

Pariza, Michael. "Japanese-Style Fermented Soy Sauce Contains an Anticancer Agent." Paper presented at the American Chemical Society's Symposium on Carcinogens, Mutagens, and Anticarcinogenic Factors in Foods, Washington, DC, April 12, 1989.

Pennington, Jean, and Helen Church. *Food Values of Portions Commonly Used*. New York: Harper & Row, 1985.

Persky, Victoria, and Linda Van Horn. "Epidemiology of Soy and Cancer: Perspectives and Directions." Paper presented at The First International Symposium on the Role of Soy in Preventing and Treating Chronic Disease, Mesa, AZ, February 20–23, 1994.

Peterson, G., and S. Barnes. "Genistein and Biochanin A Inhibit the Growth of Human Prostate Cancer Cells But Not Epidermal Growth Factor Receptor Tyrosine Autophosphorylation." *Prostate* 22, 4 (1992): 335–45.

Peterson, Greg. "Evaluation of the Biochemical Targets of Genistein in Tumor Cells." Paper presented at The First International Symposium on the Role of Soy in Preventing and Treating Chronic Disease, Mesa, AZ, February 20–23, 1994.

Potter, Susan, et al. "Depression of Plasma Cholesterol in Men by Consumption of Baked Products Containing Soy Protein." *American Journal of Clinical Nutrition* 58 (1993): 501–6.

Potter, Susan. "Overview of Proposed Mechanisms for the Hypocholesterolemic Effect of Soy." Paper presented at The First International Symposium on the Role of Soy in Preventing and Treating Chronic Disease, Mesa, AZ, February 20–23, 1994.

Present Knowledge in Nutrition. 5th edition. Washington, D.C.: The Nutrition Foundation, Inc., 1984.

Rao, A. V., and M. K. Sung. Paper presented at The First International Symposium on the Role of Soy in Preventing and Treating Chronic Disease, Mesa, AZ, February 20–23, 1994.

Rattenbury, Jeanne. "Do Soyfoods Stop the Stork?" *Vegetarian Times* (September 1995): 28.

Rinzler, Carol Ann. *The Complete Book of Food.* New York: World Almanac, 1987.

Rosenstein, D. L., R. J. Elin, J. M. Hosseini, G. Grover, and D. R. Rubinow. "Magnesium Measures Across the Menstrual Cycle in Premenstrual Syndrome." *Biological Psychiatry* 35, 8 (April 15, 1994): 557–61.

Shamsuddin, Abulkalam. "Inositol Phosphates Have Novel Anticancer Function." Paper presented at The First International Symposium on the Role of Soy in Preventing and Treating Chronic Disease, Mesa, AZ, February 20–23, 1994.

Schaefer, Ernst, et al. "Changes in Plasma Lipoprotein Concentrations and Composition in Response to a Low-Fat, High-Fiber Diet Area Associated with Changes in Serum Estrogen Concentrations in Premenopausal Women." *Metabolism* 44, 6 (June 1995): 749–56.

Schwartz, George. *Food Power.* New York: McGraw-Hill, 1979.

Schweigerer, L., and T. Fotsis. "Angiogenesis and Angiogenesis Inhibitors in Pediatric Diseases." *European Journal of Pediatrics* 151, 7 (July 1992): 472–76.

Sirtori, Cesare, et al. "Soy and Cholesterol Reduction: Clinical Experience." Paper presented at The First International Symposium on the Role of Soy in Preventing and Treating Chronic Disease, Mesa, AZ, February 20–23, 1994.

Slavin, Joanne. "Dietary Fiber: Mechanisms or Magic on Disease Prevention?" *Nutrition Today* (November/December 1990): 6–10.

Sojka, J. E., and C. M. Weaver. *Nutrition Review* 53, 3 (March 1995): 71–74.

Soybeans: Unlocking the Secret to Good Nutrition. Soybeans: How a Little Bean Becomes an Ingredient in Thousands of Products from Margarine to Tofu to Chicken Feed. Brochure. St. Louis, MO: United Soybean Board.

Stedman's Medical Dictionary. 25th edition. Baltimore, MD: Williams & Wilkins, 1990.

Steele, Vernon, Michael Pereira, Caroline Sigman, and Gary Kelloff. "Cancer Chemoprevention Agent Development Strategies for Genistein." Paper presented at The First International Symposium on the Role of Soy in Preventing and Treating Chronic Disease, Mesa, AZ, February 20–23, 1994.

"Study Finds New Evidence That Diet High in Vegetables and Grains May Protect Against Colon Cancer." American Cancer Society release, Atlanta, GA, October 6, 1992.

Tanaka, H., et al. "Metabolic Fates of Carbon Skeletons of Methionine, Serine, and Alanine in Growing Rats Fed Soybean Protein Diets." *Journal of Vitaminology* 40, 6 (December 1994): 535–46.

Thomas, Paul, ed. *Improving America's Diet and Health. Report of the Committee on Dietary Guidelines Implementation.* Washington, D.C.: National Academy Press, 1991.

Thun, Michael. "Aspirin Use and Reduced Risk of Fatal Colon Cancer." *New England Journal of Medicine* 325, 23 (December 5, 1991): 1644–46.

Traganos, F., et al. "Effects of Genistein on the Growth and Cell Cycle Progression of Normal Human Lymphocytes and Human Leukemia MOLT-4 and HL-60 Cells." *Cancer Research* 52, 22 (November 15, 1992): 6200–208.

Troll, Walter. "Prevention of Cancer by Agents that Suppress Production of Oxidants." Paper presented at the 204th American Chemical Society National Meeting, Washington, D.C., August 23, 1992.

Tsai, A. C., A. I. Vinik, A. Lasichak, and G. S. Lo. "Effects of Soy Polysaccharide on Postprandial Plasma Glucose, Insulin, Glucagon, Pancreatic Polypeptide, Somatostatin, and Triglyceride in Obese Diabetic Patients." *American Journal of Clinical Nutrition* 45, 3 (March 1987): 596–601.

U. S. Department of Agriculture. *Agriculture Handbook no. 8.* (1986).

Verschuren, W. M., et al. "Serum Total Cholesterol and Long-Term Coronary Heart Disease Mortality in Different Cultures: 25-Year Follow-up of Seven-Country Study." *Journal of the American Medical Association* 274, 2 (July 12, 1995): 131–35.

Whitten, Patricia, Carole Lewis, Elizabeth Russell, and Frederick Naftolin. "Potential Adverse Effects of Phytoestrogens." Paper presented at The First International Symposium on the Role of Soy in Preventing and Treating Chronic Disease, Mesa, AZ, February 20–23, 1994.

Wilcox, Josiah, and Barbara Blumenthal. "Thrombotic Mechanisms in Atherosclerosis: Potential Impact of Soy Proteins." Paper presented at The First International Symposium on the Role of Soy in

Preventing and Treating Chronic Disease, Mesa, AZ, February 20–23, 1994.

Winter, Arthur, and Ruth Winter. *Eat Right Be Bright*. New York: St. Martin's Press, 1988.

Winter, Ruth. *A Consumer's Guide to Medicines in Food: Nutraceuticals That Help Prevent and Treat Physical and Emotional Illnesses*. New York: Crown Publishers, 1995.

———. *A Consumer's Dictionary of Medicines: Prescription, Over-the-Counter, and Herbal*. New York: Crown Publishers, 1993.

———. *A Consumer's Dictionary of Food Additives*. 4th edition. New York: Crown Publishers, 1994.

Zarcone, R., G. Cardone, and P. Bellini. "Role of Magnesium in Pregnancy." *Panminerva Medicine* 36, 4 (December 1994): 168–70.

Index

Conversion Chart
EQUIVALENT IMPERIAL AND METRIC MEASUREMENT

American cooks use standard containers, the 8-ounce cup and a tablespoon that takes exactly 16 level fillings to fill that cup level. Measuring by cup makes it very difficult to give weight equivalents, as a cup of densely packed butter will weigh considerably more than a cup of flour. The easiest way therefore to deal with cup measurements in recipes is to take the amount by volume rather than by weight. Thus the equation reads: *1 cup = 240 ml = 8 fl. oz.   ½ cup = 120 ml = 4 fl. oz.*

It is possible to buy a set of American cup measures in major stores around the world.

In the States, butter is often measured in sticks. One stick is the equivalent of 8 tablespoons. One tablespoon of butter is therefore the equivalent to ½ ounce/15 grams.

SOLID MEASURES

U.S. and Imperial Measures		Metric Measures	
ounces	pounds	grams	kilos
1		28	
2		56	
3½		100	
4	¼	112	
5		140	
6		168	
8	½	225	
9		250	¼
12	¾	340	
16	1	450	
18		500	½
20	1¼	560	
24	1½	675	
27		750	¾
28	1¾	780	
32	2	900	
36	2¼	1000	1
40	2½	1100	
48	3	1350	
54		1500	1½
64	4	1800	
72	4½	2000	2
80	5	2250	2¼
90		2500	2½
100	6	2800	2¾

OVEN TEMPERATURE EQUIVALENTS

Fahrenheit	Celsius	Gas Mark	Description
225	110	¼	Cool
250	130	½	
275	140	1	Very Slow
300	150	2	
325	170	3	Slow
350	180	4	Moderately
375	190	5	
400	200	6	Moderately Hot
425	220	7	Fairly Hot
450	230	8	Hot
475	240	9	Very Hot
500	250	10	Extremely Hot

LIQUID MEASURES

Fluid ounces	U.S.	Imperial	Milliliters
	1 teaspoon	1 teaspoon	5
¼	2 teaspoons	1 dessertspoon	10
½	1 tablespoon	1 tablespoon	14
1	2 tablespoons	2 tablespoons	28
2	¼ cup	4 tablespoons	56
4	½ cup		110
5		¼ pint or 1 gill	140
6	¾ cup		170
8	1 cup		225
9			250
10	1¼ cups	½ pint	280
12	1½ cups		340
15		¾ pint	420
16	2 cups		450
18	2¼ cups		500
20	2½ cups	1 pint	560
24	3 cups		675
25		1¼ pints	700
27	3½ cups		750
30	3¾ cups	1½ pints	840
32	4 cups or 1 quart		900
35		1¾ pints	980
36	4½ cups		1000
40	5 cups	2 pints or 1 quart	1120
48	6 cups		1350
50		2½ pints	1400
60	7½ cups	3 pints	1680
64	8 cups or 2 quarts		1800
72	9 cups		2000